THE EASY SUPERFOODS COOKBOOK

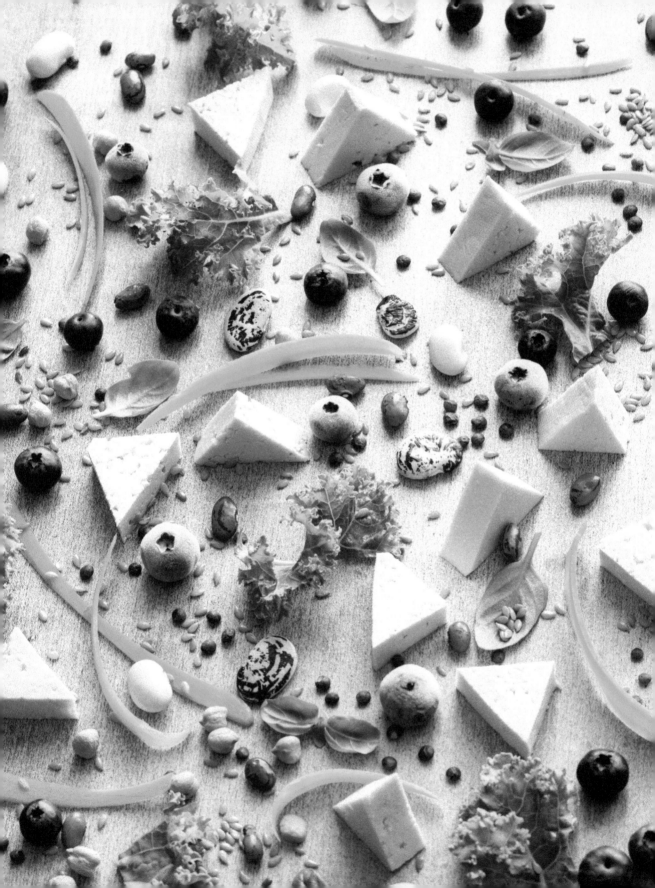

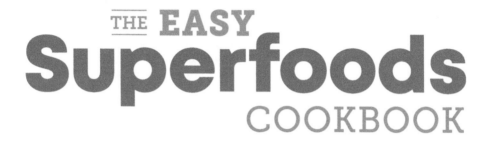

THE EASY Superfoods COOKBOOK

75 Fuss-Free, Nutrition-Packed Recipes

EMILY COOPER, RD

ROCKRIDGE PRESS

Interior and Cover Designer: Julie Gueraseva
Art Producer: Michael Hardgrove
Editor: Sam Eichner
Production Editor: Ashley Polikoff
Photography: Photography © 2019 Evi Abeler. Food styling by Albane Sharrard, cover, pp. 8, 18, 30, 40, 56, 74, 90, 104; Nadine Greeff, pp. ii, x, 116; Victoria Wall Harris, p. ix; Marija Vidal, p. vi; Helene Dujardin, p. xii; Lucia Loiso, p. 13.

ISBN: Print 978-1-64152-920-4 | eBook 978-1-64152-921-1
R0

To those who think you can't, you can.

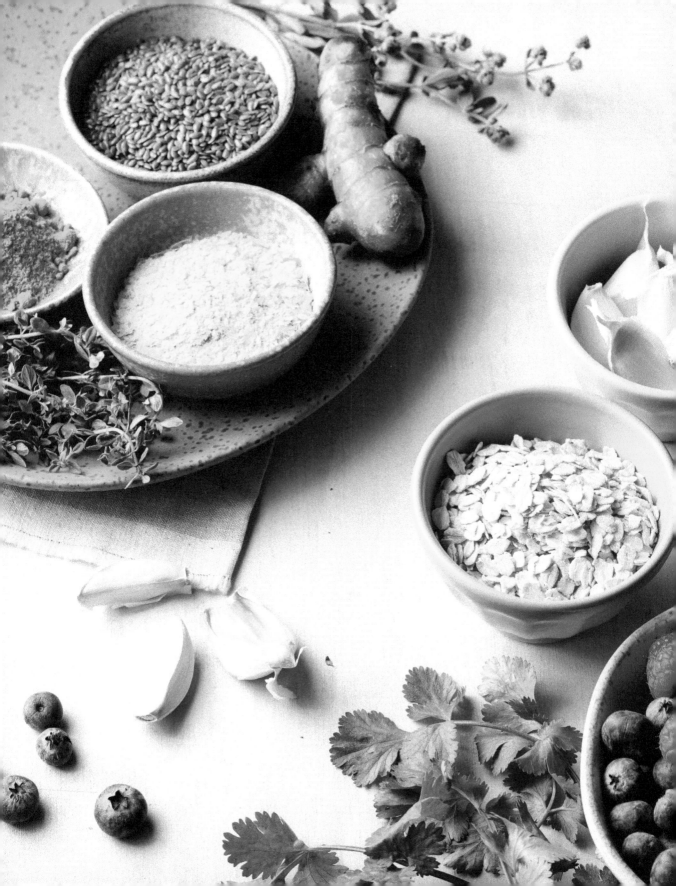

Contents

INTRODUCTION **XI**

CHAPTER 1: SUPER EASY, SUPER HEALTHY SUPERFOODS **1**

CHAPTER 2: SMOOTHIES **19**

Refreshing Watermelon-Mint Smoothie **20**

Citrus-Strawberry Smoothie **21**

Lemony Blueberry-Basil Smoothie **22**

Creamy Pineapple-Cilantro Smoothie **23**

Super Green Smoothie Bowl **24**

Vanilla Matcha Latte Smoothie **25**

Cold Brew Mocha Smoothie **26**

Triple Berry Kefir Smoothie **27**

Chocolate-Covered Cherry Smoothie **28**

Sweet Potato Pie Smoothie **29**

CHAPTER 3: BREAKFASTS **31**

Spicy Black Bean and Avocado Overnight Oats **32**

Golden Milk Oatmeal with Toasted Pecans **33**

Pumpkin-Spiced Buckwheat Pancakes **34**

Roasted Root Vegetable Hash **35**

Quinoa Breakfast Power Bowls **36**

Spinach and Artichoke Frittata **38**

CHAPTER 4: SOUPS, SALADS, AND SIDES **41**

Miso Soup with Bok Choy and Tofu **42**

Spicy Sesame Chicken Noodle Soup **43**

Creamy Avocado and Split Pea Soup **44**

Curry Vegetable Peanut Stew **45**

One-Pot Three-Bean Chili **46**

Turkey-Pumpkin Chili **47**

Sweet Corn Clam Chowder **48**

Pomegranate-Broccoli Salad **49**

Thai Sweet Potato Salad **50**

Grilled Romaine Chickpea Caesar Salad **51**

Crunchy Bok Choy Slaw **52**

Blackened Salmon Taco Salad **53**

Maple-Dijon Sautéed Kale **54**

Baked Radishes with Balsamic Vinegar **55**

CHAPTER 5: VEGETARIAN AND VEGAN ENTRÉES 57

Summer Vegetable Lasagna with Tofu Ricotta **58**

Creamy Butternut Squash and Kale Linguine **60**

Mushroom, Kale, and Farro Risotto **61**

Autumn Lentil Farro Bowls **62**

Spinach, Walnut, and Goat Cheese–Stuffed Portobello Mushrooms **63**

Ricotta, Blackberry, and Arugula Flatbreads **64**

Spinach and Feta Chickpea Burgers **65**

Spicy Peanut-Tofu Collard Wraps **66**

Tofu Spaghetti Squash Pad Thai **68**

Sweet Potato and Black Bean Burritos **70**

Roasted Red Pepper and White Bean Shakshuka **71**

Lentil-Walnut Tacos **72**

Tempeh Taco Bowls **73**

CHAPTER 6: SEAFOOD AND POULTRY 75

Gremolata-Stuffed Tilapia **76**

Ginger-Sesame Tuna Lettuce Wraps **77**

Pistachio-Crusted Salmon **78**

Coconut-Lime Shrimp Tacos **79**

Pan-Seared Scallops over Lemon-Basil Farro **80**

Grilled Chicken with Pineapple-Avocado Salsa **81**

Arugula and Goat Cheese–Stuffed Chicken Breasts **82**

Crispy Pecan-Baked Chicken **83**

Shredded Pesto Chicken Quinoa Bowls **84**

Greek Turkey and Barley–Stuffed Peppers **86**

Pineapple Curry Turkey Burgers **88**

One-Pot Turkey Pasta Primavera **89**

CHAPTER 7: BEEF AND PORK 91

Orange and Sriracha Pork Tacos 92

Bánh Mì Pork Farro Bowls 93

Oven-Roasted Pork Chops with Apples and Walnuts 94

Garlic-Herb Pork and Swiss Chard Pasta 95

Baked Tzatziki Pork Loin 96

Beef, Mushroom, and Sweet Potato Cottage Pie 97

Steak, Kale, and Goat Cheese Quesadillas 99

Beef-Stuffed Eggplant 100

Thai Basil Beef–Stuffed Sweet Potatoes 101

Mongolian Beef and Bok Choy Quinoa Bowls 102

Spinach Caprese Beef Burgers 103

CHAPTER 8: SNACKS AND DESSERTS 105

Super Seedy No-Bake Energy Bites 106

Savory Nori Popcorn 107

Grilled Chili-Lime Watermelon Wedges 108

Savory Chickpea, Feta, and Arugula Yogurt Bowl 109

Ginger Matcha "Nice" Cream 110

Trail Mix Cookies 111

Raspberry-Coconut Oatmeal Bars 112

Chocolate, Strawberry, and Avocado Mousse 114

Peanut Butter–Stuffed Baked Apples 115

MEASUREMENT CONVERSIONS 117

RESOURCES 118

REFERENCES 119

RECIPE INDEX 120

INDEX 122

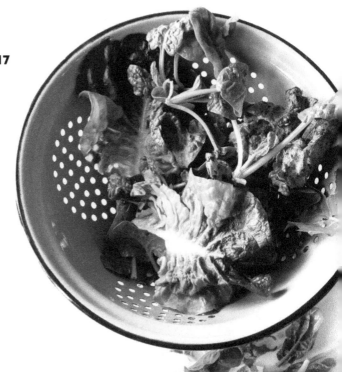

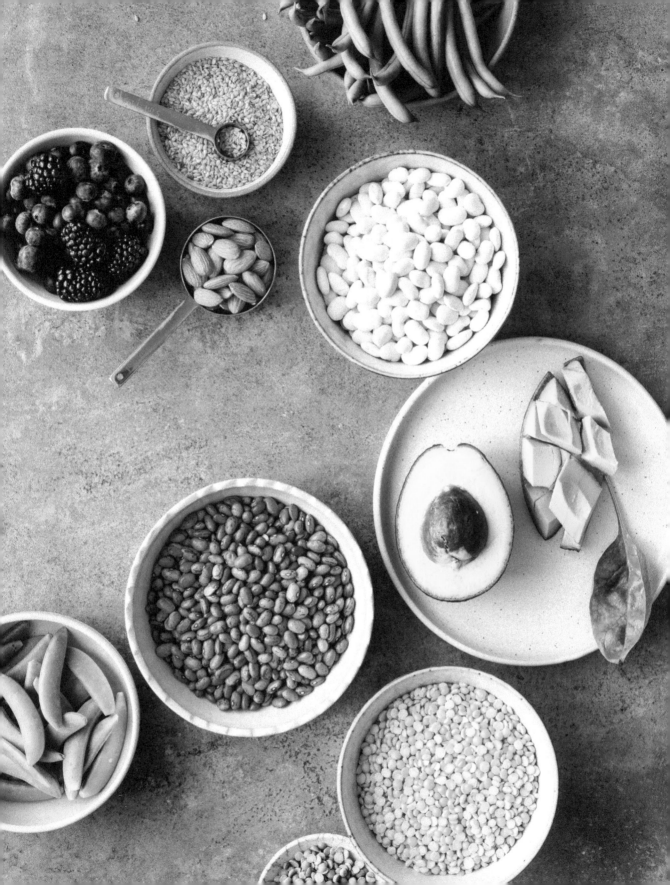

Introduction

When you hear the word "superfood," what's the first thing that comes to mind? Goji berries? Açaí? Chia seeds?

Too often, the term gets lumped in with exotic ingredients that are expensive and hard to find. In reality, superfoods aren't all that mysterious—they're simply foods with a high density of nutrients.

The Easy Superfoods Cookbook is designed to show you how to reap the health benefits of these nutrient-packed superfoods without having to spend your hard-earned money on costly and inaccessible ingredients. My hope is for you to discover that everyday items like carrots, walnuts, and spinach are just as full of supercharged nutrition as the specialty products that typically soak up the spotlight.

My interest in both a healthy lifestyle and cooking constantly inspires me to find new ways to make nutritious food taste amazing and share it with the masses—one plate at a time. It's why I became a registered dietitian in the first place. Since earning my bachelor's degree in nutrition, I've practiced in multiple areas of dietetics and launched a website, Sinful Nutrition (SinfulNutrition.com), where I share quick, easy, and nutritious recipes designed for people cooking on a budget. I've found that combining delicious dishes with good-for-you ingredients leaves me feeling more energized, more satisfied, and generally happier. It's my mission to help you feel that way, too.

Each and every recipe in this book was conceived to make eating healthier incredibly simple and, most importantly, extremely tasty! Almost all of the ingredients can be found at your local supermarket. If a recipe calls for a specialty item, I'll always provide a more readily available and affordable alternative. There are no complicated cooking techniques or special equipment required to make these dishes, either. This book makes it easy for you to become the master of preparing, cooking, and enjoying a variety of—for lack of a better word—*super* delicious and inventive superfood dishes.

So what are you waiting for? Let's get started!

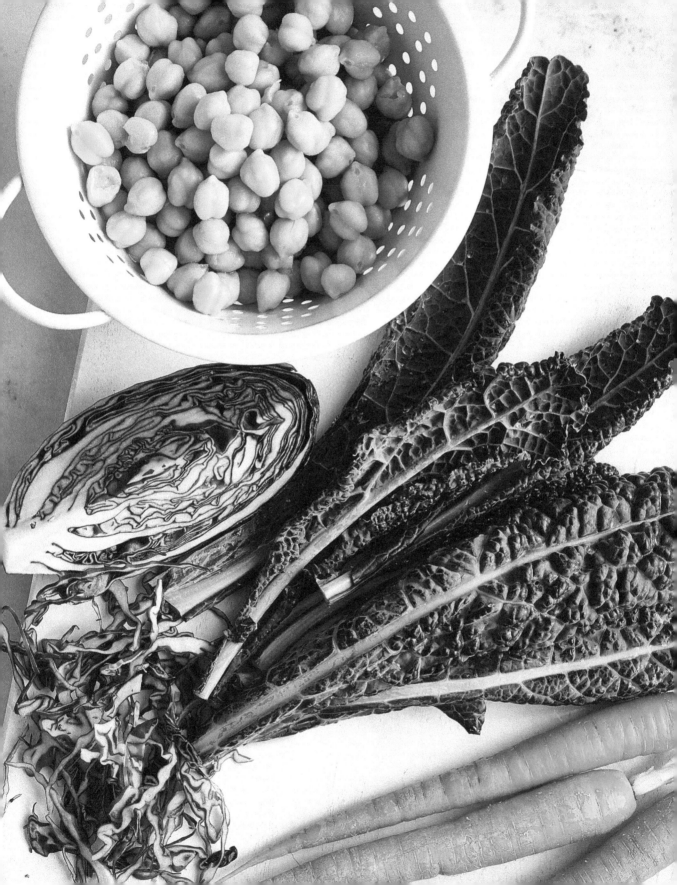

1

Super Easy, Super Healthy Superfoods

Superfoods are ingredients that everyone can and should enjoy, including you and your family! Some cookbooks or recipes may call for expensive, exotic, and hard-to-find ingredients or scare you off with a list of lengthy and complex preparation steps. The result? You end up with a bigger hole in your pocket (and schedule) than you thought. In this chapter, I'll show you that most superfoods can be found lining the shelves of your local grocery store and don't require a hefty price tag or an entire day of preparation to enjoy.

What Are Superfoods?

While there is no one-size-fits-all definition of what a superfood is, the general consensus is that the term refers to foods with a significantly higher density of health-boosting compounds (such as antioxidants, fiber, or omega-3 fatty acids) when compared to a majority of other foods. This definition may seem pretty straightforward, but there is still some conflicting information about what it truly means to be a superfood—in part because there are many different methods designed to measure nutrient density, all of which yield varying results.

For the purposes of this book, I'm defining superfoods as those which indisputably contain higher-than-average amounts of fiber, protein, heart-healthy fats, or essential vitamins and minerals. Here's one illustrative example: In this book, several recipes call for quinoa over white rice. I consider quinoa a "superfood" because every cup contains five grams of fiber and eight grams of protein, whereas every cup of white rice contains less than one gram of fiber and four grams of protein.

THE TRUTH ABOUT SUPERFOODS

You may be wondering, "Where did the term 'superfoods' even come from?" Despite its current definition, the concept wasn't the brainchild of a dietitian or doctor. Rather, it was introduced around World War I as part of the United Fruit Company's marketing campaign to sell bananas. The word didn't take off, however, until it began appearing in medical journals, when physicians started publishing their findings about a "banana diet," which was thought to help treat celiac disease. (Of course, this was before experts identified gluten as the cause of the disease's symptoms.)

In the years since, the term has become relatively common—it's especially prevalent in discussions around trendy health foods, like hemp seeds and açaí berries. But the exotic products most often associated with superfoods aren't the only ones boasting an impressive nutrient profile. Foods that can be found at almost every grocery store or farmers' market also qualify for my superfood label.

SUPERFOODS ALONE ARE NOT ENOUGH

Despite being rich sources of essential nutrients—as in, those not produced by the body itself—consuming superfoods alone is not a magic bullet for good health. Maximizing the benefits these foods offer means incorporating them into an already balanced and active lifestyle. This includes eating a varied diet of foods like fruits, vegetables, whole grains, nuts, and seeds; staying hydrated; and exercising regularly. For some, that may be a visit to the gym; for others, that can mean a walk around the block or a day working in the garden. The bottom line is this: Eating superfoods is great. But it doesn't replace the other components necessary to maintain your overall health and well-being.

NUTRITIONAL SUPPLEMENTS MAY BE CONVENIENT, but they aren't always as beneficial to your health as nutrients you absorb as part of your diet. A 2019 study in the *Annals of Internal Medicine* found that adequate intake of certain nutrients was associated with a reduced risk of death, but only when those nutrients were obtained from food sources.

Which Foods Count as Super?

Generally speaking, a food that contains a higher-than-average concentration of beneficial nutrients can be considered super. In fact, you may be pleasantly surprised to discover that some of the snacks and ingredients you and your family already enjoy on a regular basis are actually superfoods.

SUPER FRUITS

Apples Apples are a natural source of dietary fiber, including the prebiotic fiber, pectin. Fiber helps improve and regulate digestion.

Avocados Rich in monounsaturated fats, fiber, and potassium, avocados can help improve heart health and reduce inflammation in the body.

Blackberries Not to be outdone by their bluer relatives, blackberries have an impressive eight grams of dietary fiber per cup, as well as vitamin C and potassium. These nutrients are beneficial for heart health, reducing inflammation, and protecting against certain types of cancer.

Blueberries These little guys are a powerful source of antioxidants, fiber, and vitamin C, all of which can help boost immunity and heart health and protect against certain types of cancer.

Cherries Cherries are one of the few food sources of melatonin, which can help improve both sleep duration and quality. Additionally, cherries contain potassium, an important mineral for regulating blood pressure.

Oranges This citrus fruit is full of antioxidants, such as vitamin C, beta-carotene, and lycopene. Oranges can help prevent certain cancers and chronic diseases. They also have a high water content to help satisfy hydration needs.

Pineapple This tropical fruit is a rich source of manganese, a mineral that helps the body metabolize nutrients and plays a role in bone health. Pineapple also contains bromelain, a mixture of enzymes that assists with protein digestion.

Pomegranates With an antioxidant level three times higher than green tea, pomegranates boast anti-inflammatory and cancer-preventing properties.

Strawberries Full of vitamin C, fiber, and folate, strawberries contain nutrients essential for skin integrity, cell function, and regulating weight.

Watermelon The high water content of watermelon can help meet our daily hydration needs and increase feelings of fullness. Watermelon also contains the antioxidant lycopene, which can help lower blood pressure and cholesterol levels.

SUPER NUTS AND SEEDS

Almonds Ounce for ounce, almonds are the nut highest in calcium, protein, and fiber, and are also an excellent source of vitamin E, magnesium, and manganese. Calcium, magnesium, and manganese are all important nutrients for bone health and development.

Brazil nuts One of the richest food sources of selenium, a single Brazil nut can provide 100 percent of daily selenium needs for most healthy adults. This nutrient is important for thyroid function and immunity.

Pecans A natural source of phytonutrients, dietary fiber, and more than 19 vitamins and minerals, pecans are a nutrient-dense nut. They are a good source of thiamine, a B vitamin involved in cell growth and development, as well as zinc, an essential mineral involved with the immune system.

Pistachios These bright green nuts contain heart-healthy fats and are a good source of both fiber and protein. Pistachios are an excellent source of both copper and vitamin B_6, nutrients involved in energy production and metabolism.

Pumpkin seeds Snacking on pumpkin seeds will provide you with a rich source of both muscle-building protein and iron. Iron can help fight fatigue, as well as support metabolism.

Sesame seeds These tiny, tasty seeds are a rich source of fiber and protein, as well as magnesium—a mineral that plays a role in blood glucose control and blood pressure regulation.

Walnuts One of the only nuts that contains a significant amount of plant-based omega-3s, walnuts are also a source of beneficial nutrients, such as dietary fiber, protein, and magnesium. These are important for heart health, digestion, and muscle function.

> **INCLUDING SUPER NUTS AND SEEDS** in your diet is as simple as sprinkling some on top of your oatmeal in the morning, salad or grain bowl at lunch, or roasted vegetables at dinnertime. It's a quick—and delish—way to add a nutritious boost to any dish.

SUPER GRAINS

Barley Boasting a chewy texture and nutty flavor, barley is a whole grain rich in both fiber and magnesium. Both of these nutrients play an important role in regulating blood sugar levels in the body.

Buckwheat Despite its name, buckwheat actually has no relation to wheat and is naturally gluten-free. It contains multiple heart-healthy nutrients, such as antioxidants, magnesium, and dietary fiber.

Farro This ancient wheat grain is an excellent source of niacin, a B vitamin with an important role in energy production and cellular function.

Oats Whole-grain oats are particularly rich in a soluble fiber known as beta-glucan. This type of fiber plays a unique role in helping to lower levels of LDL cholesterol—often known as the "bad" cholesterol—in the body.

Quinoa While quinoa is technically a seed, this pseudo-grain is prepared and enjoyed similarly to most grains—particularly rice. Quinoa is also one of the few plant-based foods that is a complete protein. It contains all nine essential amino acids and is naturally gluten-free.

SUPER GREENS

Arugula This peppery green vegetable is an excellent source of both vitamins A and K. It also contains calcium and potassium, minerals that play a role in nerve and muscle function in the body.

Bok choy Also known as Chinese cabbage, bok choy is a cruciferous vegetable that is rich in vitamin C and vitamin K, which can help promote faster healing.

Broccoli Studies have suggested that the group of plant compounds known as isothiocyanates, which are found in broccoli and other cruciferous vegetables, can help reduce inflammation, boost immunity, and help prevent the development of certain types of cancer.

Collard greens Another cruciferous vegetable, collard greens are also an excellent source of vitamin K—a fat-soluble vitamin integral to bone development and normal clotting of the blood. A half-cup serving of cooked collard greens contains eight times the daily recommendation for vitamin K.

Kale Much like spinach, kale is full of antioxidants, calcium, and vitamin K. It also contains a surprising three grams of protein per cup, as well as fiber to help regulate digestion.

Romaine Crunchy and low in calories, romaine lettuce contains the antioxidants vitamin A and vitamin C. These nutrients not only aid in reducing inflammation in the body, but also help protect the heart.

Spinach This popular leafy green contains several antioxidants, as well as vitamin A, calcium, iron, and vitamin K.

Swiss chard Swiss chard is an excellent source of many nutrients, including vitamins A, C, and K; magnesium; iron; and potassium. The potassium, magnesium, and calcium in Swiss chard help maintain healthy blood pressure.

Need This? Eat That

NUTRIENT	HEALTH BENEFITS	FOOD SOURCES
IRON	Supports metabolism Aids cellular function Assists hormone production Treats anemia Boosts hemoglobin Builds muscle strength Increases immunity	Lean beef Oysters Poultry Leafy green vegetables Beans and legumes Tofu Fortified cereals
VITAMIN B$_{12}$	Strengthens neurological function Supports red blood cell formation Assists DNA production	Clams Haddock Salmon Tuna Trout Yogurt Fortified cereals
VITAMIN D	Helps absorb calcium Boosts nerve function Reduces inflammation Boosts immunity Helps prevent osteoporosis	Salmon Tuna Mackerel Egg yolks Cheese Fortified dairy/dairy alternatives
CALCIUM	Promotes bone health Supports muscle function Helps nerve signaling Promotes heart health	Yogurt Cheese Milk Canned salmon Sardines Lentils Fortified foods
MAGNESIUM	Regulates blood pressure Supports blood sugar control Boosts energy production Aids muscle contraction Assists nerve function	Almonds Spinach Cashews Black beans Avocados Potatoes Yogurt

Specialty Superfoods

While the more common superfoods we've covered will make up the bulk of your grocery list, it can be fun to try some more exotic options from time to time. You never know when you'll find a new favorite!

Açaí berries Native to the Amazon region, açaí berries are rich in plant compounds called anthocyanins. These not only give the fruit its deep purple hue, but also act as powerful antioxidants, and may contain as much as 10 times as many antioxidants as blueberries.

Chia seeds These tiny seeds pack a powerful nutritional punch. They contain omega-3 fatty acids, fiber, protein, and antioxidants to boost heart health.

Flaxseed The omega-3s and fiber in flaxseed can help lower cholesterol levels and help reduce the risk for heart disease.

Goji berries These brightly colored fruits contain phytochemicals and anti-oxidants that can play a role in boosting both immunity and eye health, as well as reducing inflammation in the body.

Hemp seeds A rich source of complete protein, omega-3s, and vitamin E, hemp seeds are an easy way to add a plant-based protein and heart-healthy fats to the diet.

Matcha A potent green tea powder, matcha is estimated to contain upward of 137 percent more antioxidants than regular green tea.

Miso A paste made from fermented soybeans, miso contains probiotics that can help improve both digestion and immunity.

Spirulina These blue-green algae deliver a ton of nutrition in a small package. Most often found in the form of powder, spirulina is a high-quality protein source that also contains omega-3s, antioxidants, and B vitamins. Blend it into smoothies or shakes, bake it into healthier treats, or add to water or juice. (Although, fair warning: It has a strong earthy flavor, so a little goes a long way.)

Turmeric This bright yellow spice adds more than just flavor to dishes. It is a natural source of the compound curcumin, an antioxidant with anti-inflammatory properties that can help protect against certain cancers and chronic diseases.

SUPER ROOTS AND TUBERS

Beets These bright red root vegetables are an excellent source of folate, and also contain inorganic nitrates. These plant compounds are believed to help lower blood pressure.

Carrots In addition to containing lots of vitamin A, carrots are a good source of vitamin C, which can contribute to immunity, body tissue repair, and iron absorption.

Parsnips Parsnips are an excellent source of fiber, vitamin C, and vitamin K. They are also a good source of vitamin E, a fat-soluble vitamin with antioxidant and immunity-boosting properties.

Potatoes While this humble vegetable may not get the attention it deserves, there are plenty of essential nutrients in every spud. Potatoes are a better source of potassium than bananas and are also an excellent source of vitamin C. They also contain vitamin B_6, which plays a significant role in cognitive development.

Radishes These vegetables are small but mighty. They are a good source of the immune-boosting antioxidant vitamin C. They also contain fiber, potassium, and B vitamins.

Sweet potatoes If eaten with the skin on, a medium-size sweet potato can provide daily needs for vitamin A, a crucial nutrient for vision, immunity, and bone development. Sweet potatoes also contain dietary fiber and potassium, both of which boost heart health.

SUPER LEGUMES

Black beans As an excellent source of magnesium, iron, and thiamine, black beans provide the body with essential nutrients necessary for blood pressure regulation, hormone production, and energy metabolism.

Cannellini beans In addition to being a rich source of dietary fiber and protein, cannellini beans provide both magnesium and potassium, two minerals that are key for regulating blood pressure.

Chickpeas Also known as garbanzo beans, chickpeas are an excellent source of fiber, folate, copper, iron, and manganese—an essential trace mineral that helps the body utilize a number of vitamins, such as vitamin C, vitamin E, and choline.

Green peas Like most legumes, green peas are rich in fiber and are an excellent source of vitamin K and thiamine. The B vitamin thiamine is essential for energy production and cell function in the body.

Kidney beans One of the most commonly consumed types of beans, kidney beans are rich in fiber and B vitamins. Fiber can help regulate weight and lower blood pressure levels.

Lentils One cup of these incredibly nutritious legumes contains 90 percent of the daily recommendation for folate, almost 18 grams of protein, and 16 grams of fiber.

Peanuts Most often thought of as a nut—it *is* right there in the name—people are usually surprised to learn that the peanut is actually a legume. They are full of unsaturated fats and are a rich source of plant-based protein and biotin, an essential B vitamin that supports our metabolism.

SUPER SEAFOOD

Barramundi This mild-tasting, meaty whitefish is full of heart-healthy fats. A five-ounce portion provides nearly half the weekly amount of omega-3s recommended. These healthy fatty acids can help lower triglycerides and slow the buildup of plaque in arteries.

Clams These delicious bivalves are a lean protein source that also contains high amounts of both iron and vitamin B_{12}, which both help facilitate production of red blood cells and prevent anemia.

Mussels This surprisingly easy-to-cook shellfish provides more than 100 percent of the daily recommendation for both selenium and manganese, nutrients that contribute to antioxidant functioning in the body.

Salmon Aside from being protein-rich, salmon is one of the best food sources of essential omega-3 fatty acids.

Sardines Another great source of omega-3s, sardines also contain calcium, vitamin D, and vitamin B_{12}.

Scallops As a natural source of omega-3 fatty acids, magnesium, and potassium, scallops support overall heart health.

Shrimp A concentrated protein source, shrimp is also one of the richest food sources of iodine. This is an important mineral for thyroid function and brain health.

Tuna One of the most commonly consumed seafood sources, tuna is rich in nutrients like vitamin D and selenium.

> **WHY INCLUDE HEALTHY FATS** as part of your diet? They help with cellular structure, brain and nervous system function, and nutrient absorption, among other things. Reap these benefits by eating avocados, olives, olive oil, walnuts, chia seeds, hemp seeds, salmon, and sardines.

OTHER SUPERFOODS

Eggs A whole egg contains more than 13 essential nutrients, such as choline, riboflavin, and selenium. Eggs contain antioxidants, lutein, and zeaxanthin, which have been linked to slowing the progression of age-related macular degeneration.

Ginger Often used as a spice, ginger gets its potent flavor from natural oils, especially gingerol. This compound has potent anti-inflammatory properties, which can potentially help protect against certain types of cancer.

Greek yogurt A healthy, dairy-based source of probiotics and protein is yogurt. Greek-style yogurt has a thicker texture, provides more protein, and contains less sugar than regular yogurt.

Kefir This fermented dairy beverage is a great source of calcium, protein, and gut-healthy probiotics.

Tofu Made from soybeans, tofu is a versatile, plant-based protein source that is also rich in manganese and calcium. Both of these nutrients are key components to bone formation.

Sauerkraut and kimchi The fermentation process gives cabbage-based sauerkraut and kimchi their pungent flavor and probiotic properties that can help boost immunity and gut health. Products that are shelf-stable, or have been pasteurized, kill off all types of bacteria, including the potentially beneficial probiotics. So it is best to opt for a refrigerated, unpasteurized sauerkraut or kimchi to reap the benefits of these gut-healthy microorganisms.

The Super Kitchen

The first step to cooking up delicious superfoods is stocking your pantry and refrigerator to create your super kitchen! Here are some must-have ingredients for you to keep on hand. With these around, you'll always be ready to whip up a supercharged meal. The best part: All of these ingredients provide a nutrition boost, go easy on your wallet, and are readily accessible at most supermarkets.

PANTRY ESSENTIALS

- Baking powder
- Baking soda
- Broth, vegetable
- Canned beans/lentils
- Canned fish
- Cocoa powder
- Cornstarch
- Garlic
- Honey
- Maple syrup
- Nuts and seeds (walnuts, pistachios, pumpkin seeds, chia seeds, etc.)
- Oats, rolled
- Oil, canola
- Oil, olive
- Pasta, whole-grain
- Peanut butter, natural
- Quinoa
- Rice, brown
- Tomato paste
- Vanilla extract
- Vinegar, apple cider
- Vinegar, balsamic

REFRIGERATOR AND FREEZER ESSENTIALS

- Almond milk (or your preferred dairy milk or nondairy alternative)
- Berries, frozen
- Cheese, Parmesan
- Chicken breasts, frozen
- Edamame, shelled, frozen
- Eggs
- Mustard, Dijon
- Salad greens
- Shrimp, frozen
- Spinach, frozen
- Whole fruits (apples, oranges, etc.)
- Yogurt, plain Greek

Not Quite Superfoods

While these foods don't fully qualify for superfood status, they are still healthy options that deserve a place in your grocery cart.

Bananas This perfectly portable fruit is a rich source of potassium, an essential mineral that plays an important role in fluid regulation and cell function.

Brown rice A whole grain, brown rice contains slightly higher amounts of fiber, vitamins, and minerals than white rice.

Cantaloupe A cup of this orange-hued melon contains 100 percent of the daily recommendation for vitamin C and is composed of about 90 percent water.

Celery A hydrating vegetable, celery is a rich source of vitamin K, an essential nutrient for blood clotting and bone health.

Cucumbers Relatively low in calories and high in water content, cucumbers contain dietary fiber, which can help regulate digestion and benefit gut health.

Garlic An easy way to add lots of flavor to dishes with minimal calories and sodium is with garlic. Some research has shown that high amounts of garlic may help improve immunity and heart health and lower blood pressure.

Grapes All types of grapes are natural sources of phytonutrients called polyphenols, which can contribute to heart health. They are also a rich source of vitamin K.

Macadamia nuts The macadamia nut contains monounsaturated fats and fiber, both of which can help lower cholesterol and protect against heart disease.

Sunflower seeds A handful of these is an excellent source of vitamin E and selenium, both of which function as antioxidants in the body and can help protect against certain chronic diseases.

SPICE RACK

- Cayenne
- Chili powder
- Cinnamon
- Cumin
- Curry powder
- Garlic powder

- Ginger
- Italian seasoning
- Nutmeg
- Oregano
- Paprika, smoked
- Peppercorns

- Pumpkin pie spice
- Red pepper flakes
- Salt
- Taco seasoning
- Thyme
- Turmeric

ADD SOME OF MY FAVORITE no-prep superfood snacks to your family's repertoire: a handful of almonds and an orange, apple slices spread with peanut butter and sprinkled with cinnamon, baby carrots and hummus, or a bowl of yogurt topped with walnuts and berries.

HOW TO SHOP

Now that you know the superfoods and ingredients to look for, you need to know how best to shop for them. Here are a few strategies I deploy to save time—and money—at the grocery store.

- **Check for sales.** When you're thinking of which superfoods to include for the week ahead, take a look at your grocery store flyer to see which items are on sale. This can help you decide which superfood recipes to make, and save you money in the process.

- **Make a list.** Whether it's with pen and paper or on your phone, make a list of what you need to buy. And don't forget to bring it with you!

- **Write down recipes.** When making a grocery list, I find it helpful to also list the recipes I'm planning on making. That way, if you forget why you're buying corn tortillas or an unusual spice, your recipe list will remind you. Plus, you'll see which ingredients can be used in multiple recipes.

- **Map it out.** Write out your grocery list based on how you shop. Do you hit the produce aisle first? Put your fresh fruits and vegetables on top of your list. Is dairy your first stop? Put milk, eggs, and yogurt at the top. This will keep you from running back and forth to different aisles if items are written out of order.

- **Buy in bulk.** When buying superfoods like grains, nuts, and seeds, utilize the bulk section of your grocery store. The prices are often cheaper, and these ingredients will stay fresh for a long time, especially when stored in the freezer. Utilizing the bulk section also allows you to buy just the amount you need for a recipe, instead of buying too much and having it go to waste.

ESSENTIAL EQUIPMENT

To whip up the recipes in this book, you'll want to have these common kitchen tools on hand.

Baking sheets These workhorses will be put to use for all your baking and roasting.

Blender Surprise! They're not just for smoothies. Blenders can also be used to make soups, dressings, and sauces.

Chef's knife This type of knife is both versatile and easy to control, allowing for simpler and safer chopping, slicing, and dicing.

Cutting boards Try to have at least two available. Keeping a cutting board for raw meat, poultry, and seafood and a separate one for fresh fruits and vegetables reduces the risk for cross-contamination and foodborne illnesses.

Instant-read thermometer This helpful gadget makes it easy to tell if meat, poultry, and seafood are cooked to the proper temperature.

Measuring cups and spoons Make sure you have both a liquid measuring cup and a set of dry measuring cups, since volumes can differ between solids and liquids.

Mixing bowls A set of different-size mixing bowls is helpful when making multiple dishes or a recipe with multiple components, like a dry mix and wet mix.

Pots and pans Having a set of pots and pans is essential to any kitchen.

Rubber spatula This handy tool is especially helpful for scraping down the sides of bowls or mixing ingredients in a pan without worrying about scratching it.

NICE-TO-HAVE EQUIPMENT

While these tools aren't essential, they'll make cooking superfoods—and the superfood recipes in this book—a whole lot easier. Using them may even inspire you to try new dishes and techniques.

Food processor This kitchen tool can make chopping and puréeing super quick and easy.

High-powered blender That extra speed helps take smoothies to the next level, so that what you whip up at home is as yummy as the pricey smoothie you can pick up in a shop. High-powered blenders are also great for making homemade nut butters, blended soups, and pesto.

Immersion blender Using a handheld blender, you can quickly and easily purée soups and sauces directly in the cooking pot.

Outdoor grill There's nothing like taking your cooking outdoors, especially when you want that smoky flavor added to burgers and other char-grilled meats.

Slow cooker or pressure cooker These cooking vessels are convenient for those times you want dinner to be ready when you walk through the door or on hot days when you don't want to heat up the entire kitchen.

About the Recipes

Now that we've talked about the basics, we're ready to jump into the best part: the recipes. Whether you're new to the idea of eating superfoods or looking for fresh ways to incorporate them into your already healthy diet, these easy-to-make recipes are for you. All of the dishes we'll cover are nutritious, family-friendly, and delicious.

As I mentioned earlier, the superfoods I use are readily available, so everyone can enjoy them for the healthy rock stars they truly are. Specialty items like chia seeds and seaweed will also make an appearance—after all, they're a fun way to give your meals a nutritious twist—but whenever they are featured, you can expect to find a totally accessible alternative ingredient as well. This means you can make an amazing dish with whatever superfoods work for you, your budget, and your preferences.

All of the recipes will adhere to one or more of the following categories:

5-Ingredient Recipes with this label use no more than five ingredients (not counting basics such as salt, pepper, or cooking oil).

30 Minutes In a hurry? This indicates a recipe that takes 30 minutes or less to prep and cook, from start to finish.

Budget This label marks recipes that will help you get the most nutritional bang for your buck. Each one costs approximately $5 or less per serving, based on prices at the average American supermarket.

Gluten-Free If you can't or choose not to eat gluten, these recipes are perfect for you. Always check ingredient packaging for gluten-free labeling in order to ensure foods, especially oats, were processed in a completely gluten-free facility.

One Pot These recipes use only a single cooking vessel (pot, pan, bowl, etc.), meaning less time spent cleaning up and more time spent enjoying your food.

Vegan Recipes noted as vegan don't include any animal products at all.

Vegetarian Recipes with this label use no meat or fish.

Ready to get cooking? Prepare to rock on with your superfood self!

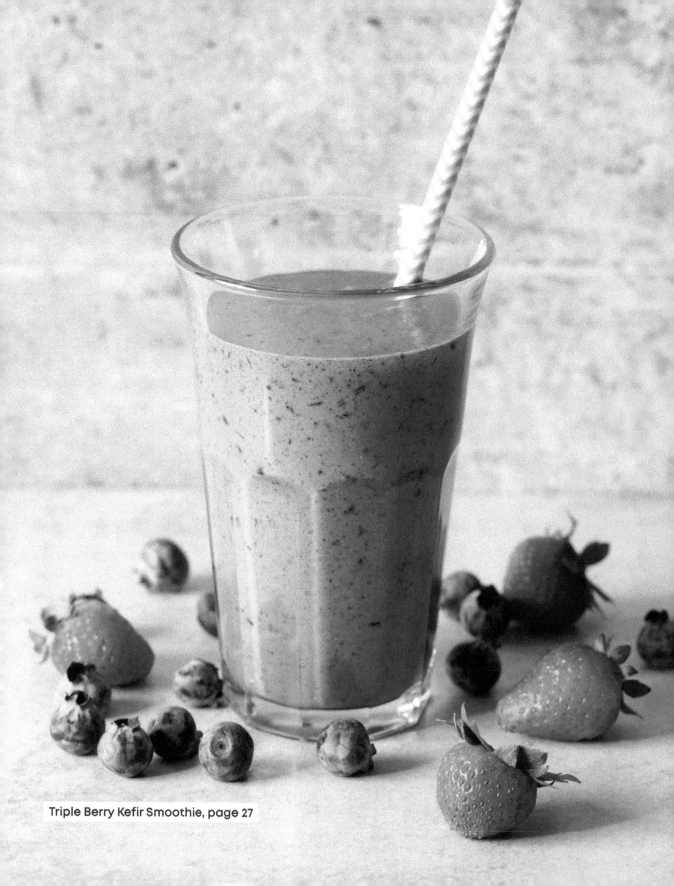

Triple Berry Kefir Smoothie, page 27

2

Smoothies

Superfood smoothies are a fast and convenient way to get loads of nutrients all in one glass. They're also perfect for getting kids and adults alike to eat more fruits and vegetables. You'll find tons of super fruits, seeds, and even vegetables in these recipes, all of which are full of antioxidants, fiber, and micronutrients to power you through the day. They each take less than 10 minutes to prepare and are easily transportable, so you can have your superfoods anytime, anywhere.

Refreshing Watermelon-Mint Smoothie

5-INGREDIENT, 30 MINUTES, GLUTEN-FREE, ONE POT, VEGAN

Prepare yourself for the ultimate refreshment in a glass. This smoothie combines the hydrating power of juicy watermelon with the cooling aura of fresh mint leaves. It is the perfect hot weather beverage—whether it's a sunny summer day or you just wish it were. A paper umbrella is optional, but strongly encouraged.

Serves: 1   **Prep time:** 5 minutes

1½ cups watermelon, diced

1 cup frozen strawberries

⅓ cup fresh mint leaves

3 tablespoons freshly squeezed lime juice

1. In a blender, combine the watermelon, strawberries, mint, and lime juice.

2. Blend on high for 1 minute, or until the mixture is completely smooth, and serve.

DID YOU KNOW? Watermelon is an excellent source of vitamin C and is higher in the antioxidant lycopene than tomatoes.

Per Serving: Calories: 143; Fat: 1g; Saturated Fat: 0g; Sodium: 13mg; Carbs: 36g; Fiber: 6g; Protein: 3g

Citrus-Strawberry Smoothie

5-INGREDIENT, 30 MINUTES, GLUTEN-FREE, ONE POT, VEGETARIAN

If you could serve sunshine in a glass, this fresh, delicious smoothie would be it. The sweet combination of strawberry and orange provides a megadose of vitamin C, which can help boost your immunity and start your day off a little bit brighter. The addition of Greek yogurt adds both protein and probiotics to satisfy your hunger and keep your gut happy.

Serves: 1   **Prep time:** 5 minutes

1 cup frozen strawberries

⅔ cup orange juice

½ cup plain, low-fat Greek yogurt

½ tablespoon hemp seeds (optional)

1. In a blender, combine the strawberries, orange juice, yogurt, and hemp seeds (if using).
2. Blend on high for 1 minute, or until the mixture is completely smooth, and serve.

SUBSTITUTION TIP: Make this smoothie vegan by replacing the Greek yogurt with silken tofu.

Per Serving: Calories: 195; Fat: 1g; Saturated Fat: 0g; Sodium: 59mg; Carbs: 35g; Fiber: 3g; Protein: 13g

Lemony Blueberry-Basil Smoothie

30 MINUTES, GLUTEN-FREE, ONE POT, VEGAN

Behold: a smoothie that's as healthy as it is refreshing. The blueberries are a natural source of antioxidants and a good source of fiber, which can aid digestion and heart health. The hemp seeds provide essential omega-3 fatty acids, which help the body absorb fat-soluble vitamins. As for the rest of the ingredients? Well, they're just here to make this drink incredibly tasty.

Serves: 1   **Prep time:** 5 minutes

1½ cups unsweetened vanilla almond milk

1 cup frozen blueberries

½ cup ice cubes

1 tablespoon grated lemon zest

2 tablespoons freshly squeezed lemon juice

1 tablespoon hemp seeds (optional)

7 fresh basil leaves

1. In a blender, combine the almond milk, blueberries, ice, lemon zest, lemon juice, hemp seeds (if using), and basil.

2. Blend on high for 1 minute, or until mixture is completely smooth, and serve.

SUBSTITUTION TIP: Not a fan of almond milk? Just use your favorite dairy milk or milk alternative instead.

Per Serving: Calories: 155; Fat: 3g; Saturated Fat: 0g; Sodium: 178mg; Carbs: 26g; Fiber: 6g; Protein: 3g

Creamy Pineapple-Cilantro Smoothie

30 MINUTES, GLUTEN-FREE, ONE POT, VEGETARIAN

If you think cilantro is just for savory dishes, it's time to think again. Pair it with juicy pineapple and lime, and you have the taste of a tropical vacation right in your glass. To make this super smoothie even creamier and more delicious, don't forget to add the heart-healthy avocado.

Serves: 1   **Prep time:** 5 minutes

1¼ cups unsweetened vanilla almond milk

1 cup baby spinach

1 cup frozen pineapple, diced

½ avocado, pitted and peeled

¼ cup fresh cilantro leaves

2 tablespoons freshly squeezed lime juice

1 teaspoon honey (optional)

1. In a blender, combine the almond milk, spinach, pineapple, avocado, cilantro, lime juice, and honey (if using).

2. Blend on high for 1 minute, or until the mixture is completely smooth, and serve.

DID YOU KNOW? An avocado a day keeps the hunger at bay! Avocados are packed with fiber and healthy fats to help keep you full longer.

Per Serving: Calories: 295; Fat: 18g; Saturated Fat: 2g; Sodium: 260mg; Carbs: 37g; Fiber: 10g; Protein: 5g

Super Green Smoothie Bowl

30 MINUTES, GLUTEN-FREE, ONE POT, VEGAN

Believe me when I say it really is this easy being green. Making your smoothie ultra-thick and spoonable is the closest you can get to eating ice cream for breakfast, albeit with the nutrient boost of fruits, vegetables, and spirulina—a blue-green algae powder packed with protein and iron.

Serves: 1   **Prep time:** 5 minutes

FOR THE SMOOTHIE

2 cups baby spinach

1 cup diced frozen mango

¾ cup unsweetened vanilla almond milk

½ cup frozen strawberries

1 teaspoon spirulina powder

FOR THE BOWL (OPTIONAL)

1 medium kiwi, peeled and sliced

¼ cup fresh blueberries

1 tablespoon unsweetened, shredded coconut

1 tablespoon goji berries

1 teaspoon chia seeds

1 teaspoon hemp seeds

TO MAKE THE SMOOTHIE

1. In a blender, combine the spinach, mango, almond milk, strawberries, and spirulina powder.

2. Blend on low for 1 minute, or until the mixture is smooth, and serve.

TO MAKE THE BOWL

Simply pour the smoothie into a bowl, and add the kiwi, blueberries, coconut, goji berries, chia seeds, and hemp seeds.

SUBSTITUTION TIP: If you prefer your smoothie bowl without spirulina, punch up the nutrition by adding an extra handful of baby spinach instead.

Per Serving: Calories: 397; Fat: 16g; Saturated Fat: 8g; Sodium: 217mg; Carbs: 61g; Fiber: 13g; Protein: 10g

Vanilla Matcha Latte Smoothie

30 MINUTES, GLUTEN-FREE, ONE POT, VEGETARIAN

Skip the long lines and make a healthier version of this coffeehouse favorite at home for a fraction of the price. Matcha is a green tea powder with a high concentration of antioxidants. The chia seeds contain heart-healthy dietary fiber and omega-3s and help give this smoothie a thicker, creamier texture.

Serves: 1   **Prep time:** 5 minutes

1 cup unsweetened vanilla almond milk

1 frozen banana

1 teaspoon matcha powder

1 teaspoon honey

1 teaspoon vanilla extract

1 teaspoon chia seeds (optional)

1. In a blender, combine the almond milk, banana, matcha powder, honey, vanilla, and chia seeds (if using).
2. Blend on high for 1 minute, or until the mixture is completely smooth, and serve.

SUBSTITUTION TIP: No matcha? No problem! Swap out half the almond milk for strong green tea that's been chilled instead.

Per Serving: Calories: 181; Fat: 3g; Saturated Fat: 0g; Sodium: 182mg; Carbs: 35g; Fiber: 5g; Protein: 3g

Cold Brew Mocha Smoothie

30 MINUTES, GLUTEN-FREE, ONE POT, VEGAN

Combine your breakfast with your morning coffee using my favorite caffeinated smoothie recipe. Cacao powder, a cold-pressed and less processed cocoa powder, adds a super-rich chocolate flavor, plus a dose of fiber and magnesium. If you don't have cold brew on hand, the same amount of chilled, strong coffee is a good substitute in this supercharged beverage.

Serves: 1 **Prep time:** 5 minutes

1 frozen banana

¾ cup black, unsweetened
cold brew coffee

¼ cup unsweetened vanilla
almond milk

1 tablespoon
cacao powder

2 teaspoons chia seeds

1 teaspoon vanilla extract

1. In a blender, combine the banana, coffee, almond milk, cacao powder, chia seeds, and vanilla.
2. Blend on high for 1 minute, or until the mixture is completely smooth, and serve.

SUBSTITUTION TIP: Regular cocoa powder works just as well as cacao powder here.

Per Serving: Calories: 315; Fat: 14g; Saturated Fat: 4g; Sodium: 51mg; Carbs: 50g; Fiber: 19g; Protein: 10g

Triple Berry Kefir Smoothie

5-INGREDIENT, 30 MINUTES, GLUTEN-FREE, ONE POT, VEGETARIAN

If you're a fan of berries, one berry just isn't enough. But three varieties of antioxidant-rich berries? I say that's just right. In this recipe, we combine these super fruits with probiotic-rich kefir to make a creamy and delicious beverage that's full of protein, fiber, and, of course, delicious berry flavor.

Serves: 1   **Prep time:** 5 minutes

1 (3½-ounce) pouch unsweetened açaí purée

1 cup plain, low-fat kefir

½ cup fresh or frozen strawberries

½ cup fresh or frozen blueberries

1. Run the pouch of açaí purée under warm water for 1 minute before opening. Pour it into a blender.
2. Add the kefir, strawberries, and blueberries.
3. Blend on high for 1 minute, or until smooth, and serve.

SUBSTITUTION TIP: Can't find açaí purée? Double the amount of blueberries used in this smoothie instead.

Per Serving: Calories: 246; Fat: 8g; Saturated Fat: 2g; Sodium: 152mg; Carbs: 34g; Fiber: 12g; Protein: 12g

Chocolate-Covered Cherry Smoothie

5-INGREDIENT, 30 MINUTES, GLUTEN-FREE, ONE POT, VEGAN

Whenever a chocolate craving hits, whip up this drinkable dessert. The chocolate and cherry combination isn't just delicious; it's also rich in antioxidants and fiber. The frozen cauliflower gives this smoothie its thick and creamy texture while seamlessly sneaking in a helping of vegetables.

Serves: 1   **Prep time:** 5 minutes

1½ cups frozen cherries

1 cup frozen
   cauliflower florets

1 cup unsweetened vanilla
   almond milk

1½ tablespoons
   cacao powder

5 ice cubes

1. In a blender, combine the cherries, cauliflower, almond milk, cacao powder, and ice.
2. Blend on high for 1 minute, or until the mixture is completely smooth, and serve.

SUBSTITUTION TIP: Don't have cacao powder? Swap it out for regular cocoa powder instead.

Per Serving: Calories: 247; Fat: 10g; Saturated Fat: 4g; Sodium: 212mg; Carbs: 48g; Fiber: 16g; Protein: 11g

Sweet Potato Pie Smoothie

30 MINUTES, GLUTEN-FREE, ONE POT, VEGETARIAN

Throw on your sweater and lace up your boots, because this smoothie is about to hit you with the taste of fall. As their name implies, sweet potatoes add a touch of natural sweetness. And they are loaded with vitamin A and potassium. I often refer to this sensational smoothie as liquid pie—and you'll soon know why.

Serves: 1   **Prep time:** 5 minutes

¾ cup unsweetened vanilla almond milk

¾ cup cooked sweet potato, mashed

1 frozen banana

½ cup plain, low-fat Greek yogurt

1 teaspoon vanilla extract

1 teaspoon maple syrup

1 teaspoon cinnamon

½ teaspoon pumpkin pie spice

1. In a blender, combine the almond milk, sweet potato, banana, yogurt, vanilla, maple syrup, cinnamon, and pumpkin pie spice.
2. Blend on high for 1 minute, or until the mixture is completely smooth, and serve.

DID YOU KNOW? Greek yogurt is rich in protein and probiotics and also adds a dose of bone-fortifying calcium.

Per Serving: Calories: 379; Fat: 3g; Saturated Fat: 0g; Sodium: 249mg; Carbs: 72g; Fiber: 10g; Protein: 17g

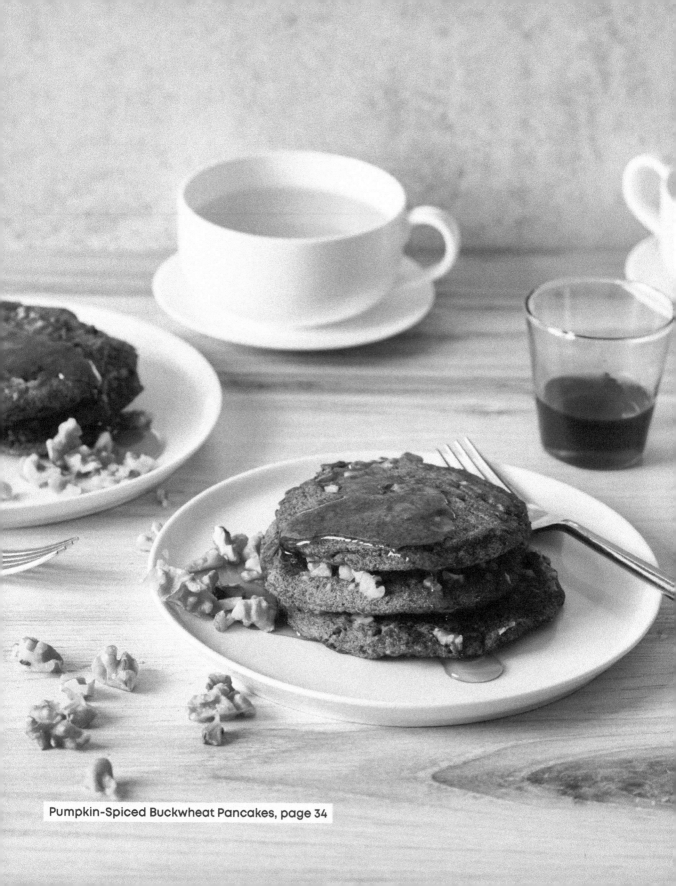

Pumpkin-Spiced Buckwheat Pancakes, page 34

3

Breakfasts

Mornings are hard. Eating a healthy breakfast shouldn't be. These yummy recipes—which feature high-protein foods like eggs and Greek yogurt and fiber-forward ingredients like walnuts and chia seeds—pack enough of a nutritional punch to prepare you for whatever the day has in store. And don't worry: Most of them can be made in less than 30 minutes, so there's no need to wake up any earlier to start your day with a nutritious meal.

Spicy Black Bean and Avocado Overnight Oats

BUDGET, VEGETARIAN

Admit it: You probably think of oatmeal as a healthy but bland breakfast. Well, these Mexican-inspired overnight oats are here to change your mind. They have black beans and oats to fill you up with fiber, avocado to provide a dose of unsaturated fats and vitamin K, and a bit of chili powder to add a hint of spice. Talk about a wake-up call!

Serves: 1   Prep time: 10 minutes, plus 4 hours to soak

¾ cup low-fat milk

½ cup rolled oats

¼ cup plain, low-fat Greek yogurt

1 teaspoon chia seeds

½ teaspoon ground cinnamon

⅓ cup canned black beans, drained and rinsed

1 teaspoon freshly squeezed lime juice

¼ teaspoon ground cumin

¼ teaspoon chili powder

¼ teaspoon garlic powder

¼ avocado, pitted, peeled, and sliced

1. In a small bowl, combine the milk, oats, yogurt, chia seeds, and cinnamon. Cover, and refrigerate for at least 4 hours or overnight.

2. Before serving, in a small microwave-safe bowl, mix together the beans, lime juice, cumin, chili powder, and garlic powder. Microwave on high for 30 seconds, or until warmed through.

3. Spoon the beans over the oats, and top with the avocado.

SERVING TIP: Like things extra spicy? Add a dash of your favorite hot sauce or cayenne before serving.

Per Serving: Calories: 447; Fat: 13g; Saturated Fat: 3g; Sodium: 124mg; Carbs: 62g; Fiber: 15g; Protein: 25g

Golden Milk Oatmeal with Toasted Pecans

30 MINUTES, BUDGET, VEGETARIAN

Consider this recipe the "golden ticket" of breakfasts. It combines the earthy flavors of a turmeric latté (also known as "golden milk") with hearty oats and toasted pecans for an all-around soul-soothing meal. If the addition of black pepper sounds odd, don't worry. It's just there to help your body absorb all the antioxidants from the turmeric.

Serves: 1   **Prep time:** 5 minutes   **Cook time:** 10 minutes

¾ cup unsweetened vanilla almond milk

½ cup rolled oats

½ teaspoon ground turmeric

½ teaspoon ground ginger

½ teaspoon ground cinnamon

½ teaspoon vanilla extract

1½ teaspoons honey

Pinch freshly ground black pepper

2 tablespoons chopped pecans

1. In a small saucepan, combine the almond milk and oats. Bring to a boil over high heat.

2. Reduce the heat to medium-low. Stir in the turmeric, ginger, cinnamon, vanilla, honey, and pepper. Cook for 5 minutes, or until the oats have thickened.

3. While the oats are cooking, heat the pecans in a small skillet over medium heat, tossing frequently to prevent scorching, for 3 minutes, or until fragrant.

4. Transfer the oatmeal to a serving bowl, and top with the pecans.

SUBSTITUTION TIP: If you want richer-tasting oats, swap out the almond milk for coconut milk.

Per Serving: Calories: 389; Fat: 15g; Saturated Fat: 2g; Sodium: 139mg; Carbs: 59g; Fiber: 7g; Protein: 8g

Pumpkin-Spiced Buckwheat Pancakes

30 MINUTES, GLUTEN-FREE, VEGETARIAN

Any time is the right time for pumpkin—and don't let anybody tell you differently. For this recipe, we're combining pumpkin with nutty and fiber-rich buckwheat flour for an extra nutrition boost. Chopped walnuts add a crunchy texture, but pumpkin seeds or dried cranberries are delicious options as well.

Serves: 2   **Prep time:** 10 minutes   **Cook time:** 15 minutes

½ cup buckwheat flour

½ teaspoon
   ground cinnamon

¼ teaspoon pumpkin
   pie spice

¼ teaspoon
   baking powder

⅛ teaspoon salt

1 large egg

½ cup pumpkin purée

½ cup unsweetened
   vanilla almond milk

½ tablespoon maple syrup

1 teaspoon vanilla extract

½ teaspoon apple
   cider vinegar

1 tablespoon
   butter, divided

½ cup chopped
   walnuts (optional)

1. In a small bowl, whisk together the flour, cinnamon, pumpkin pie spice, baking powder, and salt.

2. In a large mixing bowl, combine the egg, pumpkin purée, almond milk, maple syrup, vanilla, and vinegar.

3. To make the batter, stir the dry mixture into the wet mixture.

4. Melt 1 teaspoon of butter in a large skillet over medium-low heat.

5. Scoop ¼ cup of batter at a time into the skillet, being careful not to overcrowd the pan. Sprinkle the batter with the chopped walnuts (if using).

6. Cook the pancakes for 3 minutes, or until golden brown on the bottom; flip, and cook for 2 minutes.

7. Repeat the cooking process until all of the batter is used, coating the skillet with 1 teaspoon of butter each time before adding the batter.

SUBSTITUTION TIP: If you can't find buckwheat flour, whole-wheat flour can be used instead, but the recipe will no longer be gluten-free.

Per Serving: Calories: 250; Fat: 11g; Saturated Fat: 5g; Sodium: 203mg; Carbs: 30g; Fiber: 8g; Protein: 9g

Roasted Root Vegetable Hash

BUDGET, GLUTEN-FREE, VEGAN

Roasted vegetables, a dinnertime staple, are making a cameo at the breakfast table. This colorful twist on classic hash browns is packed with antioxidants, fiber, and vitamin A. To make mornings run more smoothly, you can either make this ahead of time and serve it at room temperature, or reheat it in a 350°F oven for 10 minutes.

Serves: 4   **Prep time:** 10 minutes   **Cook time:** 45 minutes

3 large carrots, peeled and cut into ¾-inch-thick rounds (about 2 cups)

2 medium Yukon Gold potatoes, diced (about 2 cups)

1 large bunch fresh beets, peeled and diced (about 2 cups)

1 small red onion, coarsely chopped

2 tablespoons canola oil

1½ teaspoons garlic powder

1 teaspoon salt, plus more as needed

½ teaspoon freshly ground pepper, plus more as needed

½ teaspoon dried rosemary

½ teaspoon dried oregano

1. Preheat the oven to 425°F. Line a large rimmed baking sheet with aluminum foil.

2. In a bowl, combine the carrots, potatoes, beets, onion, oil, garlic powder, salt, pepper, rosemary, and oregano. Toss until evenly coated, and transfer to the baking sheet.

3. Transfer the baking sheet to the oven, and roast, stirring halfway through, for 45 minutes, or until the vegetables are tender. Remove from the oven, and season with salt and pepper.

SERVING TIP: Serve these roasted vegetables with scrambled eggs, or mix them with lentils for a plant-powered morning meal.

Per Serving: Calories: 199; Fat: 7g; Saturated Fat: 1g; Sodium: 665mg; Carbs: 31g; Fiber: 5g; Protein: 4g

Quinoa Breakfast Power Bowls

30 MINUTES, GLUTEN-FREE, VEGETARIAN

Nothing says "power me through the day" quite like the trio of eggs, avocado, and quinoa. They provide some serious energy, thanks to the trifecta of protein, fiber, and healthy fats. If you don't have any tahini on hand, just sub in the same amount of plain or garlic hummus instead.

Serves: 2   **Prep time:** 10 minutes   **Cook time:** 15 minutes

FOR THE DRESSING

1 tablespoon
  Dijon mustard

1 tablespoon tahini
  or hummus

½ tablespoon maple syrup

½ tablespoon warm water

¼ teaspoon salt

FOR THE BOWL

1 cup water, plus
  1 tablespoon, divided

⅔ cup quinoa, rinsed

1 large sweet potato

2 teaspoons olive
  oil, divided

1 garlic clove, minced

1 bunch kale, stemmed
  and chopped
  (about 3 cups)

2 large eggs

½ avocado, pitted, peeled,
  and sliced

TO MAKE THE DRESSING

In a small bowl, whisk together the mustard, tahini, maple syrup, water, and salt.

TO MAKE THE BOWL

1. In a medium saucepan, combine the water and quinoa. Bring to a boil over high heat.

2. Reduce the heat to medium, cover, and cook for 15 minutes, or until the quinoa is tender and the water has been absorbed.

3. While the quinoa is cooking, rinse the sweet potato, and pierce with a fork. Place on a microwave-safe plate, and microwave on high for 5 to 6 minutes, or until the flesh has softened and cooked through. Dice, and set aside.

4. Heat a large skillet over medium heat.

5. Put 1 teaspoon of oil and the garlic in the pan. Cook for 30 seconds, or until fragrant.

6. Add the kale and 1 tablespoon of water. Cook for 3 to 4 minutes, or until wilted. Divide between two bowls.

7. In the same skillet, heat the remaining 1 teaspoon of oil.

8. Add the eggs, and cook for 1 minute; flip, and cook for 30 seconds, or until they are over easy.

9. Divide the eggs between the bowls, and add the sweet potato and avocado. When the quinoa is ready, divide between the bowls.

10. Drizzle with the dressing, and serve.

SUBSTITUTION TIP: Make this dish vegan by swapping out eggs for beans, cooked tofu, or tempeh.

Per Serving: Calories: 579; Fat: 24g; Saturated Fat: 4g; Sodium: 559mg; Carbs: 73g; Fiber: 12g; Protein: 22g

Spinach and Artichoke Frittata

30 MINUTES, BUDGET, GLUTEN-FREE, VEGETARIAN

Getting your fill of vegetables first thing in the morning is about to get a whole lot easier. This frittata takes a classic party dip and turns it into a protein-packed breakfast. Serve it with a side of whole-grain bread or a bowl of fruit, and you'll be ready to conquer the day.

Serves: 4   Prep time: 5 minutes   Cook time: 25 minutes

8 large eggs

½ cup grated Parmesan cheese, plus ¼ cup

½ cup low-fat milk

½ teaspoon salt

¼ teaspoon freshly ground black pepper

1 teaspoon olive oil

10 ounces fresh baby spinach

1 (14-ounce) can artichoke hearts, drained and quartered

2 garlic cloves, minced

1. Preheat the oven to 425°F.

2. In a large bowl, whisk together the eggs, ½ cup of cheese, the milk, salt, and pepper.

3. In a large oven-safe skillet, heat the oil over medium heat.

4. Add the spinach, artichokes, and garlic. Cook for 5 minutes, or until the spinach has wilted. Remove from the heat.

5. Pour the egg mixture into the pan, and top with the remaining ¼ cup of cheese.

6. Transfer the pan to the oven, and bake for 20 minutes, or until the eggs have cooked through. Remove from the oven, and let sit for 5 minutes before serving.

DID YOU KNOW? Artichokes are a good source of heart-healthy fiber, vitamin C, folate, and magnesium.

Per Serving: Calories: 299; Fat: 16g; Saturated Fat: 7g; Sodium: 789mg; Carbs: 17g; Fiber: 7g; Protein: 26g

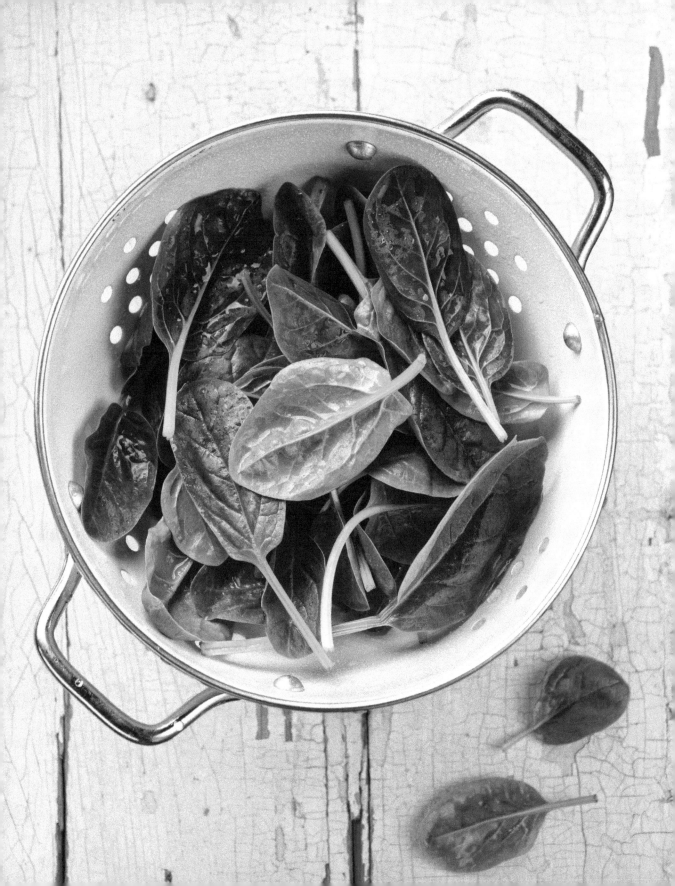

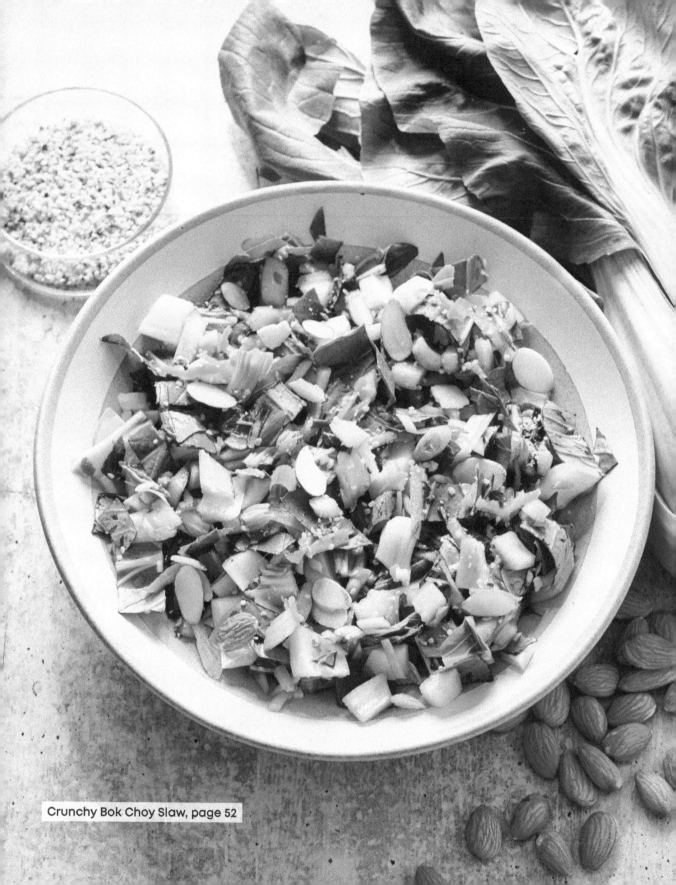

Crunchy Bok Choy Slaw, page 52

4

Soups, Salads, and Sides

Main dishes may occupy the culinary spotlight, but soups, salads, and sides can be sneaky sources of nutrition. You can expect to find an array of leafy greens, legumes, and superstar nuts and seeds in the following recipes, many of which take their cues from different cuisines around the world. Mexico, Japan, Thailand—there's no limit to where your taste buds can go with superfoods.

Miso Soup with Bok Choy and Tofu

5-INGREDIENT, 30 MINUTES, ONE POT, VEGAN

It used to be that you'd need to place an order from your favorite sushi place to enjoy this comforting soup. But now you can make it right at home—and in less time than it would take for delivery. The best part: It's made with super nutritious miso paste and vitamin C–packed bok choy.

Serves: 4   **Prep time:** 5 minutes   **Cook time:** 10 minutes

4 cups water

2 tablespoons white miso paste

2 cups chopped bok choy

¼ (14-ounce) package firm tofu, drained and finely diced

1 sheet roasted nori seaweed, roughly chopped (optional)

½ cup thinly sliced scallions

1. In a medium saucepan, bring the water to a simmer over medium-high heat.

2. Whisk in the miso paste until completely dissolved.

3. Stir in the bok choy, and cook for 5 minutes, or until softened and wilted.

4. Reduce the heat to low. Stir in the tofu, nori (if using), and scallions. Remove from heat, and serve.

DID YOU KNOW? Both miso and nori can often be found in the international aisle of your grocery store. And if you can't find bok choy, use fresh baby spinach instead.

Per Serving: Calories: 30; Fat: 1g; Saturated Fat: 0g; Sodium: 395mg; Carbs: 4g; Fiber: 1g; Protein: 2g

Spicy Sesame Chicken Noodle Soup

30 MINUTES, ONE POT

Is there anything more comforting than a bowl of chicken noodle soup? I don't think so. This twist on the classic gets a spicy makeover, which is sure to warm your belly. You can also make it vegetarian by swapping out the chicken for tofu and replacing the chicken broth with a vegetable broth.

Serves: 4   **Prep time:** 10 minutes   **Cook time:** 15 minutes

½ tablespoon canola oil

1 red bell pepper, chopped

1 yellow onion, chopped

2 large carrots, peeled and chopped

3 garlic cloves, minced

2 tablespoons grated fresh ginger

8 cups chicken broth

3 tablespoons soy sauce

2 tablespoons vinegar

1 tablespoon honey

1 tablespoon freshly squeezed lime juice

½ teaspoon red pepper flakes

6 ounces buckwheat soba noodles, broken in half

2 cups chopped cooked chicken breast

1 tablespoon sesame oil

¼ cup chopped scallions

2 teaspoons sesame seeds (optional)

1. Heat the oil in a large stockpot over medium-high heat.
2. Add the bell pepper, onion, and carrots. Cook for 5 minutes, or until softened.
3. Stir in the garlic and ginger. Cook for 30 seconds, or until fragrant.
4. Increase the heat to high. Add the broth, soy sauce, vinegar, honey, lime juice, and red pepper flakes. Bring to a boil.
5. Add the soba noodles, and cook for about 6 minutes, or until tender. Remove from the heat.
6. Stir in the chicken, sesame oil, and scallions. Serve topped with sesame seeds (if using).

SUBSTITUTION TIP: Whole-wheat spaghetti can always be used instead of soba noodles.

Per Serving: Calories: 397; Fat: 10g; Saturated Fat: 2g; Sodium: 1423mg; Carbs: 47g; Fiber: 4g; Protein: 28g

Creamy Avocado and Split Pea Soup

BUDGET, GLUTEN-FREE, ONE POT, VEGAN

The most surprising thing about this soup is that it tastes incredibly creamy but doesn't actually contain any cream. Avocado gives the soup its velvety texture—not to mention an added dose of heart-healthy fats and fiber. The split peas are a protein-rich legume, making this soup even more satisfying.

Serves: 4   **Prep time:** 10 minutes   **Cook time:** 40 minutes

1 teaspoon canola oil

1 small yellow
   onion, chopped

2 garlic cloves, minced

1 large carrot, chopped

1 celery stalk, chopped

1 bay leaf (optional)

½ teaspoon dried thyme

½ teaspoon salt

¼ teaspoon freshly ground
   black pepper

4 cups vegetable broth

1 cup split peas, rinsed

½ cup water

1 tablespoon freshly
   squeezed lemon juice

1 avocado, pitted, peeled,
   and diced

1. Heat a large stockpot over medium-high heat, and pour in the oil.

2. Stir in the onion, garlic, carrot, and celery. Cook for 5 minutes, or until softened.

3. Stir in the bay leaf (if using), thyme, salt, and pepper. Cook for 30 seconds, or until fragrant.

4. Increase the heat to high. Add the broth, split peas, and water. Bring to a boil.

5. Reduce the heat to medium-low, and simmer for 30 minutes, or until the peas have softened. Remove from the heat.

6. Add the lemon juice and avocado. Remove the bay leaf. Using an immersion blender, blend the soup in the pot until the avocado is incorporated. If the soup is too thick, add extra water.

SUBSTITUTION TIP: If you don't own an immersion blender, add half the soup to a regular blender, cover the lid with a towel, and blend on high until smooth. Then pour this purée back into the remaining soup.

Per Serving: Calories: 289; Fat: 9g; Saturated Fat: 1g; Sodium: 459mg; Carbs: 42g; Fiber: 18g; Protein: 15g

Curry Vegetable Peanut Stew

30 MINUTES, GLUTEN-FREE, ONE POT, VEGAN

Putting peanut butter in stew is popular in West African cuisine. In this recipe, it creates an unexpectedly creamy texture while tempering the spice of the curry powder. Add spinach and sweet potato for a satisfying meal brimming with beta-carotene—a precursor to vitamin A that supports eye health and immunity.

Serves: 4 **Prep time:** 10 minutes **Cook time:** 20 minutes

1 teaspoon olive oil

1 medium red onion, chopped

1 green bell pepper, chopped

1 large carrot, peeled and chopped

3 garlic cloves, minced

1 tablespoon curry powder

¼ teaspoon salt

¼ teaspoon freshly ground black pepper

1 medium sweet potato, chopped

1 bay leaf (optional)

1 (15-ounce) can diced tomatoes, drained

4 cups low-sodium vegetable broth

1½ cups frozen shelled edamame, thawed

¼ cup natural creamy peanut butter

1 (10-ounce) package frozen leaf spinach, thawed

1. In a large pot, heat the oil over medium-high heat.
2. Add the onion, bell pepper, and carrot. Cook for 3 to 4 minutes, or until slightly softened.
3. Stir in the garlic, curry powder, salt, and pepper. Cook for 1 minute, or until fragrant.
4. Add the sweet potato, bay leaf (if using), tomatoes, and broth. Increase the heat to high, and bring to a boil.
5. Reduce the heat to low, and simmer for 8 minutes, or until the sweet potato is tender.
6. Stir in the edamame, peanut butter, and spinach. Remove from the heat, remove the bay leaf, and serve.

SUBSTITUTION TIP: If you'd prefer, you can use a can of drained and rinsed chickpeas instead of edamame.

Per Serving: Calories: 366; Fat: 17g; Saturated Fat: 3g; Sodium: 329mg; Carbs: 36g; Fiber: 11g; Protein: 24g

One-Pot Three-Bean Chili

GLUTEN-FREE, ONE POT, VEGAN

The secret ingredient to a richer, heartier chili is probably not what you think it is. Surprise, it's chocolate! Yes, the addition of cacao powder—a less processed form of antioxidant-rich cocoa powder—in this satisfying, meatless chili provides a unique depth of flavor.

Serves: 4   **Prep time:** 10 minutes   **Cook time:** 25 minutes

2 teaspoons canola oil

1 green bell
pepper, chopped

1 small yellow
onion, chopped

1 large carrot, peeled
and chopped

3 garlic cloves, minced

2 tablespoons chili powder

1 tablespoon cacao powder

2 teaspoons ground cumin

1 teaspoon paprika

1 teaspoon dried oregano

½ teaspoon salt

¼ teaspoon freshly ground
black pepper

1 (6-ounce) can
tomato paste

1 (28-ounce) can
diced tomatoes

1 (15-ounce) can kidney
beans, drained and rinsed

1 (15-ounce) can black
beans, drained and rinsed

1 (15-ounce) can pinto
beans, drained and rinsed

½ cup frozen corn

2 cups water

1. Heat a large stockpot over medium heat, and pour in the oil.
2. Add the bell pepper, onion, carrot, and garlic. Cook for 5 minutes, or until softened.
3. Stir in chili powder, cacao powder, cumin, paprika, oregano, salt, and pepper. Cook for 30 seconds, or until fragrant.
4. Increase the heat to high. Add the tomato paste, diced tomatoes, kidney beans, black beans, pinto beans, corn, and water. Bring to a boil.
5. Reduce the heat to medium-low, and simmer for 15 minutes before serving. Season with salt and pepper.

SUBSTITUTION TIP: If you don't have cacao powder handy, regular cocoa powder will achieve a similar effect.

Per Serving: Calories: 424; Fat: 6g; Saturated Fat: 1g; Sodium: 402mg; Carbs: 78g; Fiber: 26g; Protein: 24g

Turkey-Pumpkin Chili

30 MINUTES, GLUTEN-FREE, ONE POT

Pumpkin may be best known for flavoring pies and lattés, but it has a savory side, too. This super quick chili is extra satisfying, thanks to the protein power of the ground turkey and the fiber from the beans and vegetables. The pumpkin adds a burst of vitamins A and C as well.

Serves: 4   **Prep time:** 5 minutes   **Cook time:** 25 minutes

1 teaspoon canola oil

1 small yellow
    onion, chopped

2 garlic cloves, minced

1 red bell pepper, chopped

1 jalapeño pepper, seeded
    and chopped

1 pound lean
    ground turkey

2½ teaspoons
    ground cumin

1 teaspoon chili powder

1 teaspoon dried oregano

1 teaspoon salt

½ teaspoon freshly ground
    black pepper

1 (15-ounce) can
    pumpkin purée

2½ cups chicken broth

1 cup frozen corn

1 (15-ounce) can pinto
    beans, drained
    and rinsed

1. Heat the oil in a large stockpot over medium heat.
2. Add the onion, garlic, bell pepper, and jalapeño pepper. Cook for 1 to 2 minutes, or until fragrant.
3. Add the ground turkey, and cook for 5 to 6 minutes, or until browned.
4. Stir in the cumin, chili powder, oregano, salt, and pepper. Cook for 30 seconds, or until fragrant.
5. Increase the heat to high. Add the pumpkin purée and chicken broth. Bring to a boil.
6. Reduce the heat to medium-low, and simmer for 5 minutes, or until the chili starts to thicken.
7. Add the corn and beans. Cook for 5 minutes, or until warmed through. Remove from the heat, and serve.

DID YOU KNOW? Red bell peppers are one of the richest sources of vitamin C. In fact, they contain more of this immune-boosting nutrient than oranges.

Per Serving: Calories: 372; Fat: 11g; Saturated Fat: 1g; Sodium: 456mg; Carbs: 35g; Fiber: 8g; Protein: 36g

Sweet Corn Clam Chowder

30 MINUTES, BUDGET, ONE POT

What happens when you merge clam chowder with corn chowder? You get a thick, twice-as-tasty soup, which you'll find yourself craving all summer and beyond. A super seafood, clams are not only a lean source of protein but also an excellent source of iron and vitamin B_{12}.

Serves: 4   **Prep time:** 10 minutes   **Cook time:** 15 minutes

½ tablespoon butter

1 small yellow onion, diced

1 celery stalk, chopped

1 garlic clove, minced

½ tablespoon
  all-purpose flour

2 cups whole milk

2 medium Yukon Gold
  potatoes, diced

¼ teaspoon dried thyme

2 ears fresh corn, husked

2 (6½-ounce) cans
  chopped clams

1 scallion, green and white
  parts, sliced

Salt

Freshly ground
  black pepper

1. In a large stockpot over medium heat, melt the butter.

2. Add the onion, and cook for 3 minutes, or until translucent.

3. Add the celery, garlic, and flour. Cook, stirring frequently, for 30 seconds, or until the garlic is fragrant.

4. Reduce the heat to medium-low. Add the milk, potatoes, and thyme. Simmer, stirring occasionally, for 10 minutes, or until the chowder starts to thicken.

5. Meanwhile, cut the corn kernels off the cobs.

6. Add the chopped clams with their juices, corn, and scallion to the pot. Remove from the heat, and season with salt and pepper.

SUBSTITUTION TIP: To make this chowder gluten-free, replace the flour with a gluten-free all-purpose flour.

Per Serving: Calories: 243; Fat: 7g; Saturated Fat: 3g; Sodium: 326mg; Carbs: 40g; Fiber: 6g; Protein: 9g

Pomegranate-Broccoli Salad

GLUTEN-FREE, ONE POT, VEGETARIAN

It's sweet, crunchy, and chock-full of incredibly healthy ingredients. What's not to love about this salad? The broccoli, apple, and pomegranate are full of fiber and antioxidants and add a satisfying crunch. Meanwhile, arils—the juice-filled, edible seeds of the pomegranate—provide a hint of sweetness and pop of bright red color.

Serves: 4   Prep time: 15 minutes, plus 30 minutes to chill

5 cups broccoli florets

1 large apple, chopped

½ cup low-fat, plain Greek yogurt

¼ cup mayonnaise

2 tablespoons vinegar

1 teaspoon honey

½ teaspoon salt

½ cup chopped walnuts

¼ cup pomegranate arils

1. In a large bowl, combine the broccoli and apple.
2. Stir in the yogurt, mayonnaise, vinegar, honey, and salt until combined.
3. Add the walnuts and pomegranate arils. Stir to combine. Refrigerate for at least 30 minutes, or until you're ready to serve.

SUBSTITUTION TIP: If you don't have pomegranate arils, add dried cranberries or dried cherries instead.

Per Serving: Calories: 306; Fat: 20g; Saturated Fat: 3g; Sodium: 435mg; Carbs: 25g; Fiber: 6g; Protein: 8g

Thai Sweet Potato Salad

VEGETARIAN

Nope, this isn't your grandma's potato salad—it's even better! After you taste it, you'll see why sweet potatoes and this Thai-inspired peanut sauce were made for each other. I especially love that it has more vitamin A and C and fiber than your classic potato salad. You can also make this dish vegan by switching out the honey for maple syrup or brown sugar.

Serves: 6 to 8   **Prep time:** 15 minutes, plus 30 minutes to chill   **Cook time:** 10 minutes

4 large sweet
  potatoes, diced

3 garlic cloves, minced

½ tablespoon minced
  fresh ginger

½ cup natural
  peanut butter

2½ tablespoons
  reduced-sodium
  soy sauce

2 tablespoons freshly
  squeezed lime juice

1½ tablespoons vinegar

½ tablespoon honey

¼ teaspoon red
  pepper flakes

2 to 3 tablespoons
  warm water

2 scallions, green
  and white parts,
  chopped, divided

¼ cup chopped peanuts

1. Put the sweet potatoes in a large stockpot, and cover with water. Bring to a boil over high heat, and cook for 6 to 8 minutes, or until tender but firm. Drain.

2. In a large bowl, to make the sauce, whisk together the garlic, ginger, peanut butter, soy sauce, lime juice, vinegar, honey, and red pepper flakes.

3. Add warm water a tablespoon at a time to thin the sauce.

4. Add the sweet potatoes and half the scallions. Stir to combine.

5. Top with the remaining scallions and the peanuts. Cover, and refrigerate for at least 30 minutes before serving.

SUBSTITUTION TIP: If you have a peanut allergy, use almonds and almond butter instead of peanuts and peanut butter.

Per Serving: Calories: 260; Fat: 14g; Saturated Fat: 2g; Sodium: 304mg; Carbs: 26g; Fiber: 5g; Protein: 10g

Grilled Romaine Chickpea Caesar Salad

5-INGREDIENT, 30 MINUTES, BUDGET, VEGETARIAN

Say hello to the new ingredient on the grill: romaine lettuce wedges. Charring them unlocks an unexpectedly smoky flavor and may just change the way you think about salads. For this recipe, I use chickpeas instead of the usual chicken to add a boost of heart-healthy fiber. If you don't have an outdoor grill, simply use a stovetop grill pan instead.

Serves: 4   **Prep time:** 10 minutes   **Cook time:** 5 minutes

2 romaine hearts, halved lengthwise

1 teaspoon olive oil

1 (15-ounce) can chickpeas, drained and rinsed

2 tablespoons Caesar dressing, plus more as needed

½ cup shaved Parmesan cheese

½ cup croutons

1. Place the romaine on a grill or a grill pan over high heat.

2. Drizzle the oil over the romaine, and grill for 30 seconds on each side, or until charred. Transfer to a serving platter.

3. In a small bowl, toss the chickpeas with the Caesar dressing, and spoon the mixture evenly over the romaine.

4. Sprinkle the Parmesan and croutons on top. If desired, serve with extra Caesar dressing.

SERVING TIP: For an alternative to serving this wedge-style, chop the romaine after grilling, and toss it in a large serving bowl with the chickpeas, Parmesan, and croutons.

Per Serving: Calories: 235; Fat: 8g; Saturated Fat: 2g; Sodium: 285mg; Carbs: 32g; Fiber: 5g; Protein: 14g

Crunchy Bok Choy Slaw

ONE POT, VEGETARIAN

Green cabbage isn't the only viable vegetable for a mean, green slaw. Enter bok choy, the star of this dish. This leafy green is an excellent source of fiber and vitamin C, which both promote heart health. Sliced almonds provide the crunch factor, as well as healthy fats, fiber, and protein.

Serves: 4   **Prep time:** 10 minutes, plus 30 minutes to chill

2 tablespoons vinegar

1 tablespoon reduced-sodium soy sauce

1 tablespoon freshly squeezed lime juice

½ tablespoon honey

¼ teaspoon red pepper flakes

1 small bunch bok choy, rinsed, stemmed, and chopped

1 large carrot, grated

1 garlic clove, minced

1 scallion, green and white parts, sliced

2 tablespoons sliced almonds

½ tablespoon hemp seeds

1. In a mixing bowl, whisk together the vinegar, soy sauce, lime juice, honey, and red pepper flakes.
2. Add the bok choy, carrot, garlic, and scallion. Stir to combine.
3. Stir in the almonds and hemp seeds. Refrigerate for at least 30 minutes before serving.

SUBSTITUTION TIP: If you don't have hemp seeds, sesame seeds are a great replacement.

Per Serving: Calories: 62; Fat: 2g; Saturated Fat: 0g; Sodium: 209mg; Carbs: 9g; Fiber: 2g; Protein: 3g

Blackened Salmon Taco Salad

30 MINUTES, GLUTEN-FREE

For a healthier take on tacos, I like to think outside the shell—literally. In this recipe, I plate the blackened salmon on a bed of fresh greens. The combination of spicy Cajun flavors and Mexican-inspired ingredients will be so satisfying, I promise you won't miss the shell.

Serves: 2   **Prep time:** 15 minutes   **Cook time:** 10 minutes

FOR THE SALMON

½ teaspoon paprika

½ teaspoon ground cumin

¼ teaspoon garlic powder

¼ teaspoon salt

¼ teaspoon freshly ground black pepper

2 (4-ounce) skinless salmon fillets

2 teaspoons canola oil

FOR THE SALAD

4 cups chopped romaine lettuce

1 avocado, pitted, peeled, and sliced

1 cup cherry tomatoes, halved

½ cup fresh corn

½ cup canned black beans, drained and rinsed

½ cup medium salsa

¼ cup Greek yogurt

1 scallion, green and white parts, sliced

TO MAKE THE SALMON

1. In a small bowl, to make the seasoning mixture, mix together the paprika, cumin, garlic powder, salt, and pepper.

2. Sprinkle the seasoning mixture evenly over both sides of the salmon fillets.

3. Heat a large skillet over medium-high heat, and pour in the oil.

4. Add the salmon skin-side up to the pan, and cook for 2 to 3 minutes, or until crispy; flip, and cook for 5 to 6 minutes, or until crispy and the flesh flakes easily with a fork.

TO MAKE THE SALAD

1. Divide the lettuce between two bowls. Top each with the salmon, avocado, tomatoes, corn, beans, and salsa.

2. Serve with a dollop of Greek yogurt and a sprinkle of scallions.

SUBSTITUTION TIP: If salmon is too pricey, feel free to use a different protein of your choice.

Per Serving: Calories: 511; Fat: 27g; Saturated Fat: 5g; Sodium: 432mg; Carbs: 38g; Fiber: 13g; Protein: 34g

Maple-Dijon Sautéed Kale

5-INGREDIENT, 30 MINUTES, GLUTEN-FREE, VEGAN

Kale is one of the all-time great superfoods, but it can taste too bitter depending on how it's prepared. That's why this nutrient-packed dish is an amazing way to get kale into your diet. The flavors of the apple cider vinegar, Dijon mustard, and maple syrup add a sweet and tangy taste that complements the natural bite of the kale.

Serves: 4   **Prep time:** 10 minutes   **Cook time:** 10 minutes

1 pound kale, stemmed and chopped

½ cup water

2 garlic cloves, minced

2 tablespoons Dijon mustard

2 tablespoons maple syrup

1 tablespoon apple cider vinegar

¼ teaspoon salt

1. Heat a large stockpot over medium heat, and add the kale and water, tossing to coat.

2. Cover the pot, and cook the kale for 5 minutes, or until it has cooked down to half the size.

3. Meanwhile, in a small bowl, whisk together the garlic, mustard, maple syrup, vinegar, and salt.

4. Remove the lid from the pot, and continue cooking the kale until all of the water has cooked off.

5. Toss the mustard mixture with the kale, and cook for 1 minute, or until the flavors meld. Remove from the heat, and serve.

SUBSTITUTION TIP: I prefer this dish with kale, but it's really fantastic with any type of leafy green, such as spinach, collard greens, or Swiss chard.

Per Serving: Calories: 90; Fat: 0g; Saturated Fat: 0g; Sodium: 286mg; Carbs: 20g; Fiber: 2g; Protein: 4g

Baked Radishes with Balsamic Vinegar

5-INGREDIENT, BUDGET, GLUTEN-FREE, VEGAN

If you're not a fan of radishes, you've never had them quite like this. Baking them until they're crispy and golden brown before tossing them with a bit of balsamic vinegar brings out their natural sweetness. So give this side dish a try. Who knows? Radishes just may become your new go-to vegetable.

Serves: 4   **Prep time:** 10 minutes   **Cook time:** 40 minutes

2 large bunches radishes

2 tablespoons canola oil

½ teaspoon garlic powder

½ teaspoon salt, plus more as needed

¼ teaspoon freshly ground black pepper, plus more as needed

2 tablespoons balsamic vinegar

1. Preheat the oven to 400°F. Line a large rimmed baking sheet with aluminum foil.

2. Rinse the radishes, and remove the tops and the bottom roots. Quarter them, and transfer to the prepared baking sheet.

3. Add the oil, garlic powder, salt, and pepper. Stir to coat.

4. Transfer the baking sheet to the oven, and bake for 20 minutes. Remove from the oven. Stir the radishes, return to the oven, and cook for another 20 minutes, or until golden and tender. Transfer to a bowl.

5. Add the vinegar, and toss. Season with salt and pepper.

DID YOU KNOW? Radishes are a natural source of vitamin C, fiber, and antioxidants—all of which help keep your heart healthy.

Per Serving: Calories: 68; Fat: 7g; Saturated Fat: 1g; Sodium: 298mg; Carbs: 1g; Fiber: 0g; Protein: 0g

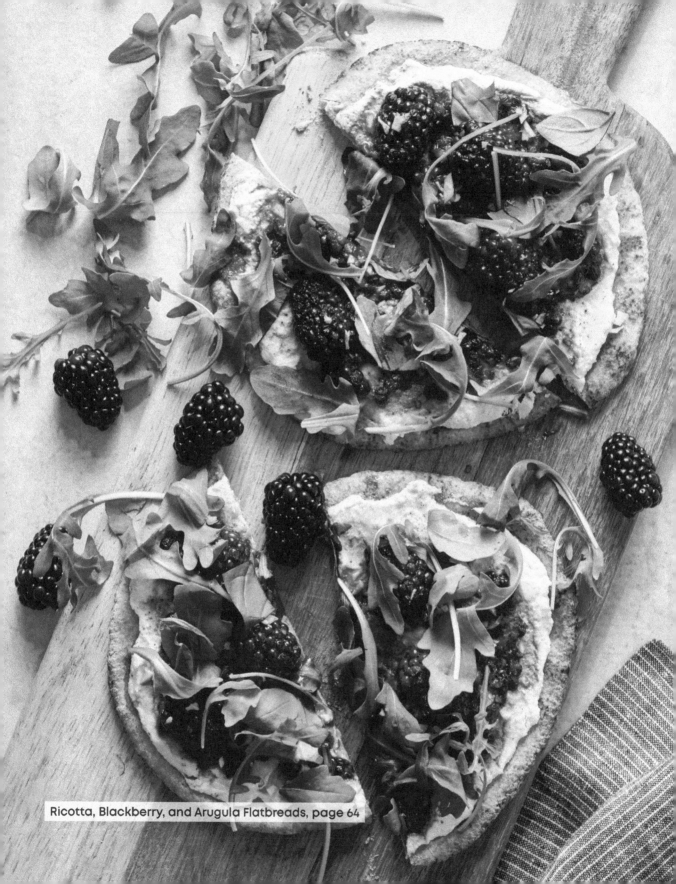

Ricotta, Blackberry, and Arugula Flatbreads, page 64

5

Vegetarian and Vegan Entrées

B ut I'm still hungry" is a common complaint lodged against the vegetarian entrées people tend to encounter. Not so with these recipes. Highlighting nutritious plant-based proteins—like tofu and lentils—the inventive, vegetable-heavy mains in this chapter are as hearty as they are healthy. Don't believe me? Just wait 'til you dig into my fabulous Spinach and Feta Chickpea Burgers.

Summer Vegetable Lasagna with Tofu Ricotta

BUDGET, VEGETARIAN

Using tofu instead of ricotta cheese may not fly in a traditional Italian kitchen, but this modern take on a classic is a big winner in my house. It tastes strikingly similar to the original but with the added benefit of more fiber and less saturated fat.

Serves: 8   **Prep time:** 15 minutes   **Cook time:** 1 hour

1 (16-ounce) package
 lasagna noodles

1 (14-ounce) package firm
 tofu, drained

1 tablespoon vinegar

½ teaspoon dried oregano

½ teaspoon salt

½ teaspoon garlic powder

2 teaspoons canola oil

3 garlic cloves, minced

1 red bell pepper,
 chopped

1 small red onion, chopped

1 medium
 zucchini, chopped

1 small eggplant, chopped

1 (10-ounce) package
 baby spinach

8 ounces sliced
 button mushrooms

3 cups marinara sauce

1 cup part-skim shredded
 mozzarella cheese,
 divided, plus 1½ cups

¼ cup grated
 Parmesan cheese

1. Preheat the oven to 350°F.
2. Cook the lasagna noodles according to the package directions, and drain.
3. In a small bowl, crumble the tofu with a fork.
4. Mix in the vinegar, oregano, salt, and garlic powder.
5. Heat a large stockpot over medium heat, and pour in the oil.
6. Add the garlic, bell pepper, onion, zucchini, and eggplant. Cook for about 8 minutes, or until softened.
7. Stir in the spinach and mushrooms. Cook for 2 minutes, or until the spinach has wilted.
8. Pour in the marinara sauce, and cook for 3 minutes, or until the mixture starts to bubble.
9. Add a spoonful of the sauce to the bottom of a 9-by-13-inch baking dish.
10. Layer the lasagna noodles over the sauce to cover the bottom of the pan.
11. Top with half the tofu mixture and ½ cup of mozzarella cheese.

12. Repeat the process one more time before adding a final layer of lasagna noodles.

13. Top with the remaining sauce, 1½ cups of mozzarella cheese, and the Parmesan cheese.

14. Cover with aluminum foil. Transfer to the oven, and bake for 40 minutes, or until the lasagna is bubbly and the cheese has melted.

15. Remove the foil, and bake for another 5 minutes, or until the cheese has browned. Remove from the oven, and let cool for 5 to 10 minutes before cutting and serving.

SERVING TIP: This recipe makes enough lasagna to serve a crowd, though if you'd rather save it all for yourself, it reheats nicely the next day, too.

Per Serving: Calories: 297; Fat: 7g; Saturated Fat: 2g; Sodium: 302mg; Carbs: 44g; Fiber: 5g; Protein: 17g

Creamy Butternut Squash and Kale Linguine

30 MINUTES, BUDGET, ONE POT, VEGAN

Believe it or not, putting together a creamy pasta dish is totally possible without butter, cheese, or cream—you just have to get creative. Using frozen puréed butternut squash cuts the prep time in half while still giving the dish its velvety texture. It is also a rich source of vitamins A and C.

Serves: 4   Prep time: 10 minutes   **Cook time:** 15 minutes

8 ounces
whole-wheat linguine

1 teaspoon canola oil

3 garlic cloves, minced

1 large bunch kale,
stemmed and chopped
(about 8 cups)

1 cup vegetable
broth, divided

20 ounces frozen
butternut squash
purée, thawed

½ teaspoon salt, plus more
as needed

¼ teaspoon freshly ground
black pepper, plus more
as needed

1 tablespoon fresh
sage, chopped

1. Cook the linguine in a medium-size pot according to the package directions and drain, transferring the linguine to a bowl nearby.

2. Using the same pot, heat the oil over medium heat.

3. Add the garlic, and cook for 30 seconds, or until fragrant.

4. Add the kale and ½ cup of broth. Cook for 3 to 5 minutes, or until the kale has wilted.

5. Reduce the heat to low. Stir in the remaining ½ cup of broth, the squash, salt, and pepper.

6. Add the linguine, and stir to combine. Season with salt and pepper.

7. Stir in the sage, and serve.

Per Serving: Calories: 347; Fat: 3g; Saturated Fat: 0g; Sodium: 555mg; Carbs: 71g; Fiber: 13g; Protein: 14g

Mushroom, Kale, and Farro Risotto

BUDGET, ONE POT, VEGETARIAN

Making a risotto may sound intimidating, but I promise it doesn't have to be. The trick is to add the broth a little bit at a time in order to achieve a rich, decadent texture. Super nutritious whole-grain farro lends the dish a pleasant hint of nuttiness. Don't be surprised if you find yourself coming back for seconds.

Serves: 4   **Prep time:** 10 minutes   **Cook time:** 40 minutes

2 teaspoons canola oil

1 small yellow onion, chopped

3 garlic cloves, minced

1½ teaspoons dried thyme

½ teaspoon salt, plus more as needed

¼ teaspoon freshly ground black pepper, plus more as needed

1 cup farro, rinsed

1 (10-ounce) package sliced button mushrooms

4 cups vegetable broth, divided

1 large bunch kale, stemmed and coarsely chopped

⅓ cup grated Parmesan cheese

1. Heat a large stockpot over medium heat, and pour in the oil.

2. Add the onion and garlic. Cook for about 3 minutes, or until the onion is translucent.

3. Stir in the thyme, salt, and pepper. Cook for 30 seconds, or until fragrant.

4. Add the farro, and cook, stirring frequently, for 1 minute.

5. Add the mushrooms and ½ cup of vegetable broth. Cook for about 3 minutes, or until all the broth has been absorbed.

6. Continue adding vegetable broth ½ cup at a time until 3 cups of broth have been used, for about 20 minutes.

7. Stir in the kale and the remaining 1 cup of broth. Cook for 4 to 5 minutes, or until the farro is tender. Remove from the heat.

8. Stir in the cheese. Season with salt and pepper.

DID YOU KNOW? Farro is an ancient grain rich in fiber, protein, and B vitamins.

Per Serving: Calories: 212; Fat: 20g; Saturated Fat: 2g; Sodium: 456mg; Carbs: 24g; Fiber: 3g; Protein: 16g

Autumn Lentil Farro Bowls

BUDGET, VEGAN

Forget pumpkin-spiced lattés—the spirit of autumn is right here in this bowl. The dressing, cinnamon, chopped apple, and dried cranberries give you the hallmark flavors of fall in every bite. If you're so inclined (and I think you will be), you can mix a batch of the dressing separately and stash it in the refrigerator to drizzle over all of your salads.

Serves: 4 **Prep time:** 10 minutes, plus overnight to soak **Cook time:** 25 minutes

FOR THE BOWLS

6 cups water

2 cups farro, soaked in water overnight

1 cup brown lentils, rinsed

1 large apple, chopped

4 cups baby spinach

2 tablespoons hemp seeds

½ cup chopped walnuts

½ cup dried cranberries

¼ cup pumpkin seeds

FOR THE DRESSING

¼ cup apple cider vinegar

3 tablespoons Dijon mustard

2 tablespoons olive oil

1 tablespoon maple syrup

1 teaspoon cinnamon

1 teaspoon salt

½ teaspoon freshly ground black pepper

TO MAKE THE BOWLS

1. In a large stockpot, bring the water to a boil.

2. Add the farro, and cook for 10 minutes, or until tender. Drain, and transfer to a large bowl.

3. Add the lentils to the pot, and cover with water. Boil, adding water to the pot as needed, for 10 to 12 minutes, or until tender. Drain, and transfer to the bowl with the farro.

4. Add the apple, spinach, hemp seeds, walnuts, cranberries, and pumpkin seeds to the bowl. Stir to combine. Divide among four bowls.

TO MAKE THE DRESSING

In a small bowl, add the vinegar, mustard, oil, maple syrup, cinnamon, salt, and pepper. Stir to combine. Distribute evenly across the four bowls, and serve.

SUBSTITUTION TIP: If you don't have hemp seeds on hand, you can mix in sunflower seeds instead.

Per Serving: Calories: 647; Fat: 27g; Saturated Fat: 3g; Sodium: 554mg; Carbs: 80g; Fiber: 12g; Protein: 25g

Spinach, Walnut, and Goat Cheese–Stuffed Portobello Mushrooms

30 MINUTES, BUDGET, GLUTEN-FREE, ONE POT, VEGETARIAN

Spinach, goat cheese, and mushrooms are one of my absolute favorite combinations, and they come together beautifully in this delicious dish. Better yet, these portobellos take almost no time to prepare but are stuffed to the brim with flavor. To turn this entrée into a crowd-pleasing appetizer, just use button mushroom caps instead of portobellos.

Serves: 4   **Prep time:** 5 minutes   **Cook time:** 15 minutes

4 large portobello mushroom caps, stemmed

1 (10-ounce) package frozen chopped spinach, thawed

2 garlic cloves, minced

6 ounces goat cheese, softened

½ teaspoon salt

¼ teaspoon freshly ground black pepper

¼ cup chopped walnuts

4 tablespoons grated Parmesan cheese, divided

1. Preheat the oven to 375°F. Line a rimmed baking sheet with aluminum foil.

2. Wipe the mushrooms with a damp towel to remove dirt and debris, and scrape out the gills with a spoon. Place upside down on the prepared baking sheet.

3. Squeeze excess water out of the chopped spinach, and put in a mixing bowl.

4. Add the garlic, goat cheese, salt, and pepper. Stir to combine.

5. Stir in the walnuts, and then divide the mixture evenly among the mushroom caps.

6. Top each mushroom cap with 1 tablespoon of Parmesan cheese.

7. Transfer the baking sheet to the oven, and bake for 12 minutes, or until the mushrooms are tender. Remove from the oven.

Per Serving: Calories: 241; Fat: 17g; Saturated Fat: 8g; Sodium: 473mg; Carbs: 9g; Fiber: 4g; Protein: 16g

Ricotta, Blackberry, and Arugula Flatbreads

30 MINUTES, BUDGET, VEGETARIAN

If you've never had fruit on a pizza before, these flatbreads are a simple and tasty place to start. I love the mix of the light flavor of the ricotta cheese, the sweetness of the berries, and the peppery bite of the arugula. The whole-wheat pita bread base is a time-saving, fiber-filled alternative to making flatbread dough.

Serves: 4   **Prep time:** 5 minutes   **Cook time:** 10 minutes

2 whole-wheat
  pita rounds

1 pint blackberries, divided

½ cup part-skim ricotta
  cheese, divided

2 garlic cloves, minced

Salt

Freshly ground
  black pepper

1 teaspoon olive oil

1 cup arugula

1 tablespoon
  chopped basil

1. Preheat the oven to 425°F. Put the pita rounds on a large baking sheet.

2. In a small bowl, smash half the blackberries with the back of a fork. Then add the remaining blackberries.

3. Spread ¼ cup of ricotta cheese onto each pita round.

4. Top with the blackberries and garlic. Season with salt and pepper.

5. Transfer the baking sheet to the oven, and bake for 8 to 10 minutes, or until the bottoms of the pitas are golden brown and crispy. Remove from the oven.

6. Drizzle with oil, and top with the arugula and basil.

7. Cut each pita round in half, and serve.

SUBSTITUTION TIP: Fresh blueberries are a perfectly good alternative to blackberries.

Per Serving: Calories: 173; Fat: 5g; Saturated Fat: 2g; Sodium: 211mg; Carbs: 27g; Fiber: 6g; Protein: 8g

Spinach and Feta Chickpea Burgers

30 MINUTES, BUDGET, VEGETARIAN

They say, "Feta is bettah," and these Greek-inspired chickpea burgers are proof. When combined with antioxidant-rich spinach and garlic, the chickpeas make these burgers just as flavorful as your standard cheeseburger. Try pairing them with baked sweet potato fries or roasted rosemary potato wedges for the full burger experience.

Serves: 4   **Prep time:** 10 minutes   **Cook time:** 10 minutes

1 (28-ounce) can chickpeas, drained and rinsed

2 tablespoons all-purpose flour

2 garlic cloves, minced

1 tablespoon freshly squeezed lemon juice

¼ teaspoon salt

¼ teaspoon freshly ground black pepper

2 cups frozen chopped spinach, thawed

⅔ cup crumbled feta cheese

2 teaspoons olive oil

4 whole-wheat hamburger buns

1. In a large bowl, using a potato masher or a fork, mash and combine the chickpeas, flour, garlic, lemon juice, salt, and pepper until most of the chickpeas are well mashed.

2. Squeeze excess water from the spinach, and stir into the chickpea mixture along with the cheese, until well combined.

3. Form the mixture into 4 patties, as you would with ground beef.

4. Heat a large skillet or sauté pan over medium heat, and add the oil.

5. Add the patties to the pan, and cook for 3 minutes on each side, or until golden brown.

6. Serve each patty on a bun, and top with any desired condiments.

SUBSTITUTION TIP: Make these burgers gluten-free by trading the regular all-purpose flour for gluten-free all-purpose flour and serving them on gluten-free hamburger buns, over greens, or in a lettuce wrap.

Per Serving: Calories: 433; Fat: 13g; Saturated Fat: 5g; Sodium: 477mg; Carbs: 62g; Fiber: 14g; Protein: 20g

Spicy Peanut-Tofu Collard Wraps

30 MINUTES, BUDGET, ONE POT, VEGAN

Here's an easy way to up your leafy green intake: Wrap protein-rich tofu, tossed in a spicy peanut sauce, in collard greens. Not only are the greens themselves healthy, but they are also a lighter, lower carbohydrate alternative to the usual tortilla wrap. And if you're like me, you'll do yourself a favor and double the amount of peanut sauce, so you'll have extra for dipping.

Serves: 4   **Prep time:** 15 minutes

FOR THE PEANUT SAUCE

½ cup natural crunchy
    peanut butter

¼ cup apple cider vinegar

¼ cup freshly squeezed
    lime juice

¼ to ½ cup water, divided

2 tablespoons
    reduced-sodium
    soy sauce

2 teaspoons brown sugar

1 teaspoon grated
    fresh ginger

½ teaspoon red
    pepper flakes

TO MAKE THE PEANUT SAUCE

In a mixing bowl, whisk together the peanut butter, vinegar, lime juice, ¼ cup of water, soy sauce, sugar, ginger, and red pepper flakes. If the sauce is too thick, add up to another ¼ cup of water, 1 tablespoon at a time.

FOR THE WRAPS

1 (14-ounce) package extra-firm tofu, drained and diced

4 large collard green leaves, stemmed

½ cucumber, sliced lengthwise

2 large carrots, grated

½ cup coleslaw mix

1 tablespoon hemp seeds

Sriracha, for serving (optional)

TO MAKE THE WRAPS

1. Add the tofu to the bowl with the peanut sauce, and toss to coat.

2. Lay the collard green leaves flat on a clean work surface, and fill evenly with the tofu.

3. Add the cucumber, carrot, and coleslaw mix to each leaf.

4. Sprinkle with hemp seeds, and drizzle with sriracha sauce (if using).

5. Fold in the sides, roll in a similar fashion to a burrito, and serve.

SUBSTITUTION TIP: Instead of hemp seeds, you can also use toasted sesame seeds.

Per Serving: Calories: 387; Fat: 24g; Saturated Fat: 4g; Sodium: 471mg; Carbs: 17g; Fiber: 6g; Protein: 25g

Tofu Spaghetti Squash Pad Thai

BUDGET, GLUTEN-FREE, VEGETARIAN

If you're looking for a healthy alternative to spaghetti, you should give spaghetti squash a try. The fiber-rich strands are perfect for soaking up this sweet-and-salty sauce, while the eggs and tofu provide a solid serving of protein. This recipe calls for tamari, a typically gluten-free Japanese soy sauce (always check the label), but if you don't need to avoid gluten, you can always use standard reduced-sodium soy sauce instead.

Serves: 4   **Prep time:** 10 minutes   **Cook time:** 50 minutes

1 large spaghetti squash, halved lengthwise and seeded

3 garlic cloves, chopped

¼ cup reduced-sodium tamari

1 tablespoon freshly squeezed lime juice

1 tablespoon brown sugar

1 teaspoon canola oil

1 (14-ounce) package firm tofu, drained and diced

3 large eggs

3 scallions, green and white parts, chopped

½ cup chopped peanuts

1. Preheat the oven to 400°F. Line a baking sheet with parchment paper or aluminum foil.

2. Place the squash cut-side down on the prepared baking sheet. Transfer to the oven, and bake for 40 minutes, or until tender. Remove from the oven. Flip, and let cool cut-side up on the baking sheet until cool enough to handle.

3. While the squash is baking, whisk together the garlic, tamari, lime juice, and sugar in a small bowl to make the sauce.

4. Heat a large skillet or sauté pan over medium-high heat, and pour in the oil.

5. Add the tofu, and cook for 5 minutes, or until browned.

6. Crack the eggs into the pan, and scramble until they are cooked through.

7. Scrape out the flesh of the squash with a fork. Add to the pan, and pour in the sauce. Stir to coat, and cook for 5 minutes, or until the sauce has thickened. Remove from the heat.

8. Top with the scallions and peanuts, and serve.

SERVING TIP: Make this dish vegan by omitting the eggs.

Per Serving: Calories: 250; Fat: 16g; Saturated Fat: 3g; Sodium: 131mg; Carbs: 19g; Fiber: 2g; Protein: 13g

Sweet Potato and Black Bean Burritos

30 MINUTES, BUDGET, GLUTEN-FREE, VEGETARIAN

Even if you're a big fan of burritos, you've probably never had one quite like this. They are made naturally gluten-free by trading out the usual tortilla for a sweet potato skin. Sweet potato skins are completely edible, full of fiber, and ideal for holding all the spicy, sweet, and protein-rich filling packed into this recipe.

Serves: 4   **Prep time:** 10 minutes   **Cook time:** 15 minutes

4 large sweet potatoes

1 tablespoon
   ground cumin

1 teaspoon chili powder

1 (15-ounce) can black
   beans, drained
   and rinsed

3 cups baby
   spinach, chopped

1½ cups frozen
   corn, thawed

1 cup salsa

1 cup shredded
   sharp Cheddar
   cheese (optional)

2 tablespoons fresh
   cilantro, chopped

1. Rinse the sweet potatoes, and pierce with a fork. Place on a microwave-safe plate, and microwave on high for 8 to 10 minutes, or until tender. Set aside until cool enough to handle.

2. Cut off one end from each sweet potato, and scoop the flesh into a large microwave-safe bowl, leaving enough flesh (about ¼ inch) intact to help them keep their shape.

3. To make the filling, mash the sweet potato flesh with the cumin and chili powder.

4. Stir in the beans, spinach, corn, salsa, and cheese (if using). Heat in the microwave for 2 minutes, or until heated through. (Alternatively, the mixture can be heated in a saucepan over medium heat.)

5. Stir the cilantro into the filling. Stuff each sweet potato skin with filling, and serve.

INGREDIENT TIP: If you have time, you can bake the sweet potatoes in the oven for 45 to 50 minutes instead of microwaving them to really bring out their sweetness and achieve a firmer texture.

Per Serving: Calories: 277; Fat: 2g; Saturated Fat: 0g; Sodium: 398mg; Carbs: 58g; Fiber: 13g; Protein: 11g

Roasted Red Pepper and White Bean Shakshuka

30 MINUTES, BUDGET, GLUTEN-FREE, ONE POT, VEGETARIAN

This simple poached egg dish, popular in Mediterranean cuisine, gets an Italian-inspired makeover with the addition of roasted red peppers, fresh basil, and garlic. The white beans in the dish give it a satisfying boost of both fiber and protein. And finishing the shakshuka with a sprinkle of salty feta cheese? That's a must.

Serves: 4   **Prep time:** 10 minutes   **Cook time:** 20 minutes

1 teaspoon canola oil

2 garlic cloves, minced

1 small yellow onion, chopped

½ teaspoon salt

½ teaspoon dried oregano

½ teaspoon dried thyme

¼ teaspoon freshly ground black pepper

1 (28-ounce) can crushed tomatoes

1 (15-ounce) can white beans, drained and rinsed

½ cup roasted red pepper strips

8 large eggs

½ cup crumbled feta cheese

2 tablespoons fresh basil, chopped

1. Heat a large skillet or sauté pan over medium heat, and pour in the oil.

2. Add the garlic and onion. Cook for 3 minutes, or until the onion is translucent.

3. Stir in the salt, oregano, thyme, and pepper. Cook for 30 seconds, or until fragrant.

4. Reduce the heat to medium-low. Add the tomatoes, and simmer for 5 to 6 minutes, or until thickened.

5. Stir in the beans and red peppers.

6. Crack the eggs into the tomato sauce, spacing them out evenly.

7. Cover the pan, and cook for 10 to 15 minutes, or until the egg whites have cooked and the yolks have set. Remove from the heat.

8. Sprinkle the cheese and basil on top, and serve.

SERVING TIP: This dish is excellent with slices of crusty whole-grain bread, which you can use to soak up all of that flavorful sauce.

Per Serving: Calories: 392; Fat: 16g; Saturated Fat: 6g; Sodium: 832mg; Carbs: 38g; Fiber: 14g; Protein: 26g

Lentil-Walnut Tacos

30 MINUTES, BUDGET, GLUTEN-FREE, ONE POT, VEGAN

Walnuts and lentils probably aren't the first ingredients you think of when it comes to tacos. But I'm about to change that. Combining the two creates a meaty texture that soaks up the savory flavor from the spices and tomato so well, they'll be a Taco Tuesday staple in no time. Bonus: The walnuts provide healthy fats to help lower cholesterol levels and support heart health.

Serves: 4   **Prep time:** 5 minutes   **Cook time:** 25 minutes

½ cup brown lentils, rinsed

1 teaspoon canola oil

2 garlic cloves, minced

1 teaspoon chili powder

1 teaspoon ground cumin

½ teaspoon smoked paprika

¼ teaspoon salt

¼ teaspoon freshly ground black pepper

1 (6-ounce) can tomato paste

½ cup water, plus more as needed

⅔ cup chopped walnuts

8 corn tortillas

1. Put the lentils in a stockpot, and cover with water. Bring to a boil over high heat. Then reduce the heat to medium-low, and simmer for 15 minutes, or until tender. Drain, and transfer to a bowl.

2. Heat the oil in the same pot over medium-high heat.

3. Add the garlic, and cook for 30 seconds, or until fragrant.

4. Stir in the chili powder, cumin, paprika, salt, and pepper. Cook for 10 seconds, or until fragrant.

5. Add the tomato paste, and stir to combine.

6. Stir in ½ cup of water, the lentils, and walnuts. Simmer for 5 minutes, or until the mixture has thickened. Add more water as needed if the mixture becomes too thick. (If you have a food processor, the mixture can be pulsed to resemble the texture of ground meat.)

7. Spoon the lentil mixture into the tortillas, and serve.

SERVING TIP: These tacos are extra delicious—and even better for you—when topped with diced avocado, cilantro, chopped tomatoes, and a squirt of freshly squeezed lime juice.

Per Serving: Calories: 381; Fat: 16g; Saturated Fat: 2g; Sodium: 222mg; Carbs: 48g; Fiber: 14g; Protein: 14g

Tempeh Taco Bowls

BUDGET, VEGAN

Tempeh is a plant-based protein made from fermented soybeans. It boasts a pleasantly firm texture and a plenty of gut-friendly probiotics. I like to toss it in a bowl with fresh vegetables, quinoa, and spicy taco seasoning for a delicious dinner or fuss-free workday lunch.

Serves: 4   **Prep time:** 10 minutes   **Cook time:** 25 minutes

2½ cups water, plus 3 tablespoons

2 cups quinoa, rinsed

1 (8-ounce) package tempeh, finely chopped

2 teaspoons taco seasoning

2 cups chopped romaine lettuce

1 avocado, pitted, peeled, and diced

1 cup frozen corn, thawed

1 red bell pepper, chopped

¼ cup chopped fresh cilantro

4 lime wedges

1. In a large stockpot, bring the water to a boil over high heat.

2. Add the quinoa, and reduce the heat to medium-low. Cover and simmer for 10 to 15 minutes, or until the water has been absorbed. Remove from the heat.

3. Put the tempeh and 2 tablespoons of water in a large skillet over medium-high heat. Cover, and cook for 5 minutes, or until the water has evaporated.

4. Remove the lid, and add the taco seasoning and the remaining 1 tablespoon of water. Cook for 3 minutes, or until fragrant.

5. Divide the quinoa evenly among four bowls, and top with the lettuce, avocado, corn, bell pepper, and tempeh.

6. Garnish with the cilantro and lime wedges, and serve.

SUBSTITUTION TIP: Making your own taco seasoning is really simple! Combine 1 tablespoon chili powder, 2 teaspoons paprika, 2 teaspoons onion powder, 1 teaspoon ground cumin, 1 teaspoon paprika, 1 teaspoon garlic powder, ½ teaspoon oregano, ½ teaspoon salt, and ¼ teaspoon freshly ground black pepper in a resealable jar.

Per Serving: Calories: 551; Fat: 19g; Saturated Fat: 3g; Sodium: 232mg; Carbs: 76g; Fiber: 11g; Protein: 25g

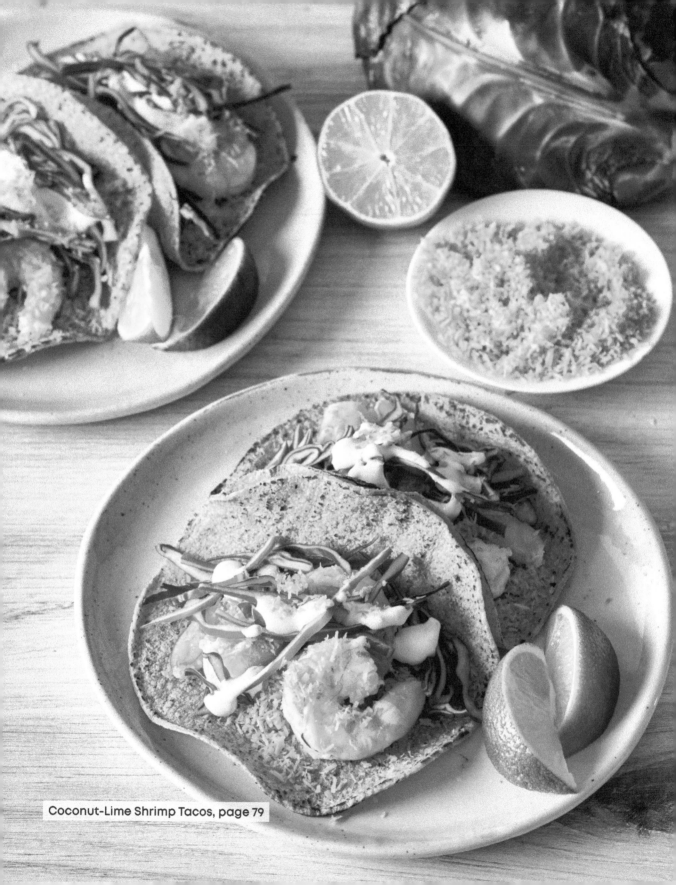

Coconut-Lime Shrimp Tacos, page 79

6

Seafood and Poultry

By incorporating nutrient-rich ingredients like fresh herbs, citrus, nuts, seeds, and garlic, these recipes will transform your everyday fish, chicken, and turkey dishes into bona fide superfood superstars. They'll also help you break out of the all-too-common food rut. With many of these dishes drawing inspiration from the cuisines of Thailand, Mexico, China, and the Mediterranean, this chapter is bringing a world of flavors right to your plate.

Gremolata-Stuffed Tilapia

5-INGREDIENT, 30 MINUTES, BUDGET, GLUTEN-FREE

Gremolata, an Italian mixture of fresh herbs, lemon, and garlic, is a natural complement to seafood. One of my favorite ways to enjoy it is as a stuffing for fish. In this recipe, I use tilapia, a mild-tasting whitefish that's both a lean source of protein and high in the immune-boosting mineral selenium. I love how the fragrant gremolata brings out the natural flavors of the fish—and you will, too!

Serves: 4   **Prep time:** 10 minutes   **Cook time:** 15 minutes

½ cup parsley,
   finely chopped

3 garlic cloves, minced

4 teaspoons grated
   lemon zest

4 (4-ounce) tilapia
   fillets, skinned

2 teaspoons olive oil

½ teaspoon garlic powder

½ teaspoon salt

¼ teaspoon freshly ground
   black pepper

1. Preheat the oven to 400°F. Line a rimmed baking sheet with parchment paper or aluminum foil.

2. In a small bowl, stir together the parsley, garlic, and lemon zest.

3. Pat the fillets dry with a paper towel, and put them on the prepared baking sheet. Spoon the parsley mixture onto one end of each fillet. Starting from the end with parsley mixture, roll up each fillet, and use toothpicks to hold in place.

4. Drizzle the fillets with the oil, and sprinkle the garlic powder, salt, and pepper on top.

5. Transfer the baking sheet to the oven, and bake for 10 to 12 minutes, or until the fillets flake easily with a fork. Remove from the oven. Remove toothpicks before serving.

SERVING TIP: This dish goes well with quinoa tossed with roasted red peppers and Italian seasoning, or roasted potatoes coated with garlic and rosemary.

Per Serving: Calories: 122; Fat: 3g; Saturated Fat: 1g; Sodium: 336mg; Carbs: 2g; Fiber: 1g; Protein: 22g

Ginger-Sesame Tuna Lettuce Wraps

30 MINUTES, BUDGET, GLUTEN-FREE, ONE POT

Your same old tuna salad is getting a long-overdue makeover. This version is protein-packed, lower in carbohydrates, and full of Asian-inspired flavor. It's a great way to utilize canned tuna, an inexpensive, natural source of protein, selenium, and omega-3 fatty acids.

Serves: 4   **Prep time:** 10 minutes

2 (6-ounce) cans white-meat tuna packed in water, drained

2 garlic cloves, minced

2 teaspoons grated fresh ginger

½ sheet nori seaweed, finely chopped

2 teaspoons freshly squeezed lime juice

1 teaspoon sesame oil

6 Bibb lettuce leaves

1 teaspoon sesame seeds, toasted

1. In a mixing bowl, flake the tuna with a fork.
2. Stir in the garlic, ginger, nori, lime juice, and oil.
3. Spoon the tuna evenly onto the lettuce leaves, and top with the sesame seeds.

SUBSTITUTION TIP: If you don't have nori seaweed, chopped scallion makes for a tasty swap.

Per Serving: Calories: 130; Fat: 2g; Saturated Fat: 0g; Sodium: 46mg; Carbs: 4g; Fiber: 0g; Protein: 23g

Pistachio-Crusted Salmon

5-INGREDIENT, 30 MINUTES, GLUTEN-FREE

This dish is one of my favorite ways to enjoy salmon, not to mention its serving of omega-3 fatty acids. Once you try this super seafood with a pistachio crust—adding a satisfying crunch and color—I'm sure it will be on your short list as well.

Serves: 4   **Prep time:** 10 minutes   **Cook time:** 15 minutes

1½ pounds skin-on salmon fillets

¼ cup salted and shelled pistachios, finely chopped

¼ cup fresh dill, finely chopped

2 teaspoons grated lemon zest

¼ teaspoon freshly ground black pepper

1. Preheat the oven to 450°F. Line a baking sheet with parchment paper.
2. Place the fillets skin-side down on the prepared baking sheet.
3. In a small bowl, combine the pistachios, dill, lemon zest, and pepper.
4. Press the pistachio mixture firmly on top of the fillets.
5. Transfer the baking sheet to the oven, and bake for 10 to 15 minutes, or until the fillets flake easily with a fork. Remove from the oven. Cut into four portions, and serve.

SERVING TIP: Serve this salmon with a side of cooked quinoa or brown rice and roasted vegetables like sweet potatoes or asparagus.

Per Serving: Calories: 216; Fat: 7g; Saturated Fat: 0g; Sodium: 241mg; Carbs: 4g; Fiber: 1g; Protein: 37g

Coconut-Lime Shrimp Tacos

30 MINUTES, GLUTEN-FREE

Prepare yourself for a one-of-a-kind coconut shrimp experience. This no-fuss recipe rivals the dishes at your favorite restaurants. Marinating the shrimp in coconut milk, lime, and garlic creates the first layer of fresh flavor. The second layer comes after they land in the corn tortillas, where you'll top them with toasted coconut, shredded red cabbage, and homemade coconut sour cream.

Serves: 4   **Prep time:** 5 minutes, plus 10 minutes to refrigerate   **Cook time:** 10 minutes

1 pound shrimp, peeled and deveined

3 garlic cloves, minced

½ cup canned coconut milk, divided

2 tablespoons grated lime zest, divided

1 tablespoon freshly squeezed lime juice

½ cup shredded coconut

¼ cup sour cream

2 teaspoons canola oil

8 corn tortillas

1 cup shredded red cabbage

8 lime wedges (optional)

1. In a large bowl, combine the shrimp, garlic, ¼ cup of coconut milk, 1 tablespoon of lime zest, and the lime juice. Cover, and refrigerate for 10 minutes.

2. Meanwhile, heat a large skillet over medium-high heat. Put the shredded coconut in the pan, and cook for 2 to 3 minutes, stirring frequently to avoid burning, until toasted and browned. Transfer to a small bowl.

3. In a separate bowl, whisk together the remaining ¼ cup of coconut milk, remaining 1 tablespoon of lime zest, and the sour cream to make the coconut sour cream.

4. Heat a skillet over high heat, and pour in the oil.

5. Remove the shrimp from the refrigerator, and use tongs to transfer them to the skillet. Discard the marinade. Cook for 2 to 3 minutes per side, or until pink and the flesh is opaque. Remove from the heat.

6. Divide the shrimp evenly among the tortillas. Top with the toasted coconut, cabbage, and coconut sour cream. Serve with lime wedges, if desired.

SERVING TIP: To switch things up, skip the tortilla, and serve the shrimp on a bed of greens or in lettuce cups instead.

Per Serving: Calories: 342; Fat: 17g; Saturated Fat: 12g; Sodium: 420mg; Carbs: 28g; Fiber: 5g; Protein: 23g

Pan-Seared Scallops over Lemon-Basil Farro

30 MINUTES

Searing scallops may seem tricky, but starting with a hot pan and not over-crowding them will deliver you that perfect, golden-brown finish. You'll be surprised by how bright and flavorful they'll taste on a bed of herbaceous, lemony farro. (To save some time, look for the pearled variety of farro. It cooks more quickly than semi-pearled.)

Serves: 4   **Prep time:** 5 minutes   **Cook time:** 25 minutes

1 cup pearled farro, rinsed

3½ cups vegetable broth

2 tablespoons fresh basil, chopped

1 teaspoon grated lemon zest

1 tablespoon freshly squeezed lemon juice

½ teaspoon garlic powder

½ teaspoon salt, plus more as needed

¼ teaspoon freshly ground black pepper, plus more as needed

1 pound sea scallops (about 16)

½ tablespoon canola oil

1. In a 6-quart stockpot, combine the farro with the vegetable broth. Bring to a boil over high heat. Reduce the heat to low, and simmer for 10 to 15 minutes, or until tender. Remove from the heat.

2. Add the basil, lemon zest, lemon juice, garlic powder, salt, and pepper. Stir to combine.

3. Heat a large skillet over medium-high heat.

4. Meanwhile, pat the scallops dry with a paper towel. Season with salt and pepper.

5. Pour the oil into the pan. Working in batches if needed to avoid overcrowding the pan, add the scallops, and cook for 2 minutes, or until golden brown. Using tongs, flip, and cook for 1 minute, or until golden brown on the other side. Remove from the heat.

6. Divide the farro among four bowls. Top with the scallops, and serve.

SUBSTITUTION TIP: For a gluten-free alternative to farro, switch to brown rice or quinoa.

Per Serving: Calories: 257; Fat: 4g; Saturated Fat: 0g; Sodium: 474mg; Carbs: 31g; Fiber: 4g; Protein: 25g

Grilled Chicken with Pineapple-Avocado Salsa

30 MINUTES, GLUTEN-FREE

Take a trip to the tropics without leaving the comfort of your own kitchen. Simple grilled chicken is anything but boring when topped with pineapple, cilantro, and lime. Diced avocado gives the salsa a creamy element, some healthy fats, and fiber. And if you don't have an outdoor grill, no problem. Just cook the chicken on your stove using a grill pan over medium heat.

Serves: 4   **Prep time:** 10 minutes   **Cook time:** 20 minutes

FOR THE SALSA

1 cup chopped pineapple

1 avocado, diced

¼ red onion, finely chopped

2 tablespoons chopped fresh cilantro

2 tablespoons freshly squeezed lime juice

Pinch cayenne (optional)

FOR THE CHICKEN

2 teaspoons canola oil

4 boneless, skinless chicken breasts

½ teaspoon salt

¼ teaspoon freshly ground black pepper

TO MAKE THE SALSA

In a small bowl, combine the pineapple, avocado, onion, cilantro, lime juice, and cayenne (if using).

TO MAKE THE CHICKEN

1. Preheat the grill on medium-high heat or a grill pan over medium heat, and coat with the oil.

2. Put the chicken on the grill, and season with the salt and pepper. Cook for 5 to 8 minutes on each side, or until an instant-read thermometer inserted into the thickest part of each breast reaches an internal temperature of 165°F. Transfer to a serving platter.

3. Spoon the salsa over the chicken, and serve.

DID YOU KNOW? Pineapple is a rich source of immunity-boosting vitamin C, with more than 100 percent of the recommended daily amount in a 1-cup serving.

Per Serving: Calories: 259; Fat: 13g; Saturated Fat: 3g; Sodium: 335mg; Carbs: 11g; Fiber: 4g; Protein: 26g

Arugula and Goat Cheese-Stuffed Chicken Breasts

5-INGREDIENT, 30 MINUTES, GLUTEN-FREE, ONE POT

This chicken is quite literally stuffed with flavor. Along with the creaminess of goat cheese, the addition of peppery arugula takes this baked chicken up a notch. And the arugula provides more than just flavor—it is also a rich source of vitamins A and K.

Serves: 4   **Prep time:** 5 minutes   **Cook time:** 20 minutes

4 boneless, skinless chicken breasts

4 ounces goat cheese

2 cups arugula

2 teaspoons canola oil

1 teaspoon Italian seasoning

½ teaspoon garlic powder

1. Preheat the oven to 400°F. Line a baking sheet with aluminum foil.

2. Put the chicken on the prepared baking sheet, and cut a pocket on the side of each breast; do not cut all the way through.

3. Fill each pocket with an equal amount of cheese and arugula.

4. Use 3 to 4 toothpicks to close up the pocket on each piece of chicken.

5. Rub the chicken with the oil, and season with the Italian seasoning and garlic powder.

6. Transfer the baking sheet to the oven, and bake for 20 minutes, or until an instant-read thermometer inserted into the thickest part of the chicken reaches an internal temperature of 165°F. Remove from the oven. Remove the toothpicks before serving.

SERVING TIP: Turn this into a complete meal by serving the chicken on a bed of quinoa with your favorite vegetables.

Per Serving: Calories: 224; Fat: 10g; Saturated Fat: 4g; Sodium: 182mg; Carbs: 1g; Fiber: 0g; Protein: 32g

Crispy Pecan-Baked Chicken

5-INGREDIENT, 30 MINUTES, GLUTEN-FREE

Many recipes rely on bread crumbs for crispiness. But not this one. The crunch factor here comes from a crust of chopped pecans, which happen to be full of healthy fats and fiber. A base of maple syrup and Dijon mustard pumps up the flavor for an all-around winner of a chicken dinner.

Serves: 4   **Prep time:** 10 minutes   **Cook time:** 20 minutes

4 boneless, skinless
   chicken breasts

2 tablespoons
   Dijon mustard

1 tablespoon maple syrup

¼ teaspoon salt

¼ teaspoon paprika

½ cup finely
   chopped pecans

1. Preheat the oven to 400°F. Line a baking sheet with aluminum foil.

2. Put the chicken on the prepared baking sheet.

3. In a small bowl, mix together the mustard, maple syrup, salt, and paprika. Spoon over the chicken.

4. Sprinkle the pecans over the chicken, and press gently to help them adhere.

5. Transfer the baking sheet to the oven, and bake for 20 minutes, or until an instant-read thermometer inserted into the thickest part of the chicken breasts reaches an internal temperature of 165°F. Remove from the oven.

SERVING TIP: Enjoy this chicken with a side of roasted or mashed potatoes.

Per Serving: Calories: 236; Fat: 12g; Saturated Fat: 1g; Sodium: 311mg; Carbs: 6g; Fiber: 2g; Protein: 28g

Shredded Pesto Chicken Quinoa Bowls

5-INGREDIENT, 30 MINUTES, GLUTEN-FREE

I often refer to this dish as "pesto presto bowls," and you'll soon understand why. These satisfying bowls come together in a flash. You can make them even faster if you have a stand mixer with a paddle attachment; simply add the chicken to the bowl and mix on medium speed until shredded.

Serves: 4   **Prep time:** 10 minutes   **Cook time:** 15 minutes

4 boneless, skinless chicken breasts

1 cup quinoa, rinsed

2 cups water

½ cup basil pesto, divided

1 cup part-skim shredded mozzarella cheese

2 cups cherry tomatoes, halved

¼ cup grated Parmesan cheese (optional)

1. Put the chicken in a large pot, and fill with enough water to cover the chicken.

2. Bring to a boil over high heat. Reduce the heat to medium-low, and simmer for 10 to 15 minutes, or until an instant-read thermometer inserted into the thickest part of the chicken breasts reaches an internal temperature of 165°F.

3. While the chicken is cooking, in a 6-quart saucepan, combine the quinoa and water. Bring to a boil over high heat. Reduce the heat to medium-low. Simmer for 10 minutes, or until all liquid is absorbed. Remove from the heat.

4. Stir in ¼ cup of pesto and the mozzarella cheese.

5. Drain the chicken, and transfer to a large mixing bowl.

6. Using two forks, shred the chicken into bite-size pieces.

7. Add the remaining ¼ cup of pesto to the bowl with the chicken, and stir to combine.

8. Divide the quinoa among four bowls. Top with the chicken and cherry tomatoes. Sprinkle with the Parmesan cheese (if using).
9. To enjoy the following day, combine any leftover chicken, quinoa, and cheese in a microwave-safe container with a lid, and place it in the refrigerator. Reheat it in the microwave for 1 to 2 minutes, and top with cherry tomatoes before serving.

DID YOU KNOW? Quinoa is full of protein and fiber and is naturally gluten-free.

Per Serving: Calories: 478; Fat: 20g; Saturated Fat: 3g; Sodium: 432mg; Carbs: 37g; Fiber: 5g; Protein: 37g

Greek Turkey and Barley–Stuffed Peppers

BUDGET

Barley is typically associated with soups, but it can do so much more. To unleash the full potential of this vitamin-rich whole grain, I like to pair it with ground turkey and ingredients like oregano, feta cheese, and chickpeas. Also known as garbanzo beans, chickpeas add a lot of protein to the mix, as well as fiber and B vitamins.

Serves: 4 **Prep time:** 10 minutes **Cook time:** 1 hour

1¾ cups water

1 cup quick-cooking barley

1 (15-ounce) can crushed tomatoes, divided

4 green bell peppers, seeded and tops removed

1 pound lean ground turkey

2 garlic cloves, minced

1 small red onion, chopped

2 teaspoons dried oregano

1 teaspoon dried thyme

1 teaspoon salt

½ teaspoon freshly ground black pepper

1 (15-ounce) can chickpeas, drained and rinsed

8 cups fresh baby spinach

½ cup crumbled feta cheese

1. In a 4-quart saucepan, bring the water to a boil over high heat.

2. Stir in the barley, reduce the heat to low, and simmer for 10 minutes, or until tender. Remove from the heat.

3. Preheat the oven to 375°F.

4. Pour ½ cup of crushed tomatoes into the bottom of an 8-inch-square baking dish.

5. Cut a thin slice off the bottom of each pepper so it can stand upright in the baking dish.

6. Put the turkey in a large skillet over medium heat, and cook for 4 to 5 minutes, or until browned.

7. Add the garlic and onion, and cook for 3 minutes, or until fragrant.

8. Stir in the oregano, thyme, salt, and pepper. Cook for 30 seconds, or until fragrant.

9. Reduce the heat to low. Stir in the chickpeas, remaining crushed tomatoes, and the spinach. Cook for 2 to 3 minutes, or until the spinach has wilted. Remove from the heat.

10. Fill the peppers with the mixture, and top with the cheese.

11. Cover the peppers tightly with aluminum foil, and place upright in the baking dish.

12. Transfer the baking dish to the oven, and bake for 30 minutes. Remove the foil, and bake for another 10 minutes, or until the peppers are tender. Remove from the oven.

SUBSTITUTION TIP: You can always swap out barley here for brown rice or quinoa, which would make this dish gluten-free.

Per Serving: Calories: 531; Fat: 8g; Saturated Fat: 3g; Sodium: 821mg; Carbs: 77g; Fiber: 17g; Protein: 45g

Pineapple Curry Turkey Burgers

5-INGREDIENT, 30 MINUTES, BUDGET, GLUTEN-FREE

This is not your average, everyday turkey burger. The Indian-inspired flavors of curry and ginger merge beautifully with the sweet caramelized pineapple packed into every juicy bite. For a better char, these burgers can also be cooked on an outdoor grill. Just make sure it's been preheated on medium-high heat.

Serves: 4   **Prep time:** 10 minutes   **Cook time:** 20 minutes

1 pound lean ground turkey

2 teaspoons finely chopped fresh ginger

2 teaspoons curry powder

2 garlic cloves, minced

½ teaspoon salt

2 teaspoons canola oil, divided

4 fresh or canned pineapple rings

1. In a large bowl, combine the turkey, ginger, curry powder, garlic, and salt.

2. Form the turkey mixture into 4 patties.

3. Heat a large skillet over medium-high heat, and pour in 1 teaspoon of oil.

4. Working in 2 batches if needed to avoid overcrowding the pan, add the patties. Cook for 6 minutes on each side, or until an instant-read thermometer inserted into the patties reaches an internal temperature of 165°F. Remove from the heat.

5. Wipe out the pan with a damp paper towel, and add the remaining 1 teaspoon of oil.

6. Add the pineapple rings, and cook for 1 to 2 minutes on each side, or until caramelized.

7. Top the patties with the pineapple before serving.

SERVING TIP: Serve these burgers on your favorite rolls, and top with a dollop of plain yogurt or sour cream, if desired.

Per Serving: Calories: 190; Fat: 4g; Saturated Fat: 0g; Sodium: 347mg; Carbs: 12g; Fiber: 2g; Protein: 29g

One-Pot Turkey Pasta Primavera

30 MINUTES, ONE POT

How do you make a hearty protein and fiber-rich pasta dish even easier to whip up? By making it all in one pot! Adding the vegetables to the pasta water during the last few minutes of cooking keeps them bright and tender, which locks in their nutrients—and spares you from washing an extra dish. I'd call that a win-win.

Serves: 4 to 6   **Prep time:** 10 minutes   **Cook time:** 20 minutes

1 (16-ounce) package whole-wheat penne

1 red bell pepper, chopped

1 medium zucchini, cut into half moons

1 small head broccoli, cut into florets

1 pound lean ground turkey

1 teaspoon salt, plus more as needed

¼ teaspoon freshly ground black pepper, plus more as needed

3 garlic cloves, minced

1 small red onion, chopped

½ cup vegetable broth

2 teaspoons grated lemon zest

1 tablespoon olive oil

½ cup grated Parmesan cheese (optional)

1. Cook the penne according to the package directions. During the last 3 minutes of cooking, add the bell pepper, zucchini, and broccoli. Drain, and transfer the penne and vegetables to a bowl.

2. Put the turkey in the same pot, and cook over medium heat for 4 to 5 minutes, or until browned. Add the salt and pepper.

3. Add the garlic and onion. Cook for 3 minutes, or until the onion has softened.

4. Add the penne, vegetables, and broth, and cook for 5 minutes, or until heated through. Remove from the heat.

5. Add the lemon zest, oil, and Parmesan cheese (if using). Toss, season with salt and pepper, and serve.

SUBSTITUTION TIP: Make this gluten-free by swapping out the whole-wheat penne for your favorite gluten-free version.

Per Serving: Calories: 627; Fat: 9g; Saturated Fat: 1g; Sodium: 511mg; Carbs: 87g; Fiber: 11g; Protein: 52g

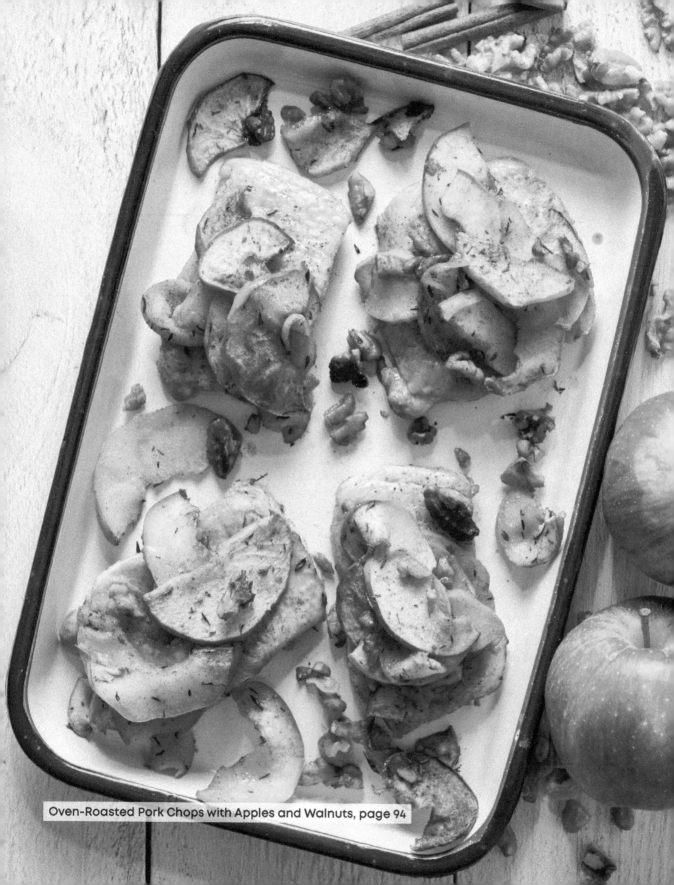

Oven-Roasted Pork Chops with Apples and Walnuts, page 94

7

Beef and Pork

I enjoy taking favorite comfort foods and infusing them with a variety of superfoods to boost the nutritional value of some of our most beloved dishes. In this chapter, you'll find colorful, nutrient-rich spins on classics such as pork chops and cottage pie, as well as unexpected flavors from Greece, Vietnam, and Italy.

Orange and Sriracha Pork Tacos

30 MINUTES, BUDGET

One taste of these tacos, and you'll know the meaning of sweet heat. The ground pork is tossed in a honey-sesame glaze spiked with sriracha. Making these tacos all in one pan helps make this dish super quick to make and clean up—meaning you'll have more time to enjoy every bite.

Serves: 4   **Prep time:** 10 minutes   **Cook time:** 10 minutes

2 garlic cloves, minced

1 teaspoon grated orange zest

½ cup freshly squeezed orange juice (about 2 large oranges)

1 tablespoon sriracha

1 tablespoon reduced-sodium soy sauce

1 tablespoon honey

½ tablespoon cornstarch

½ teaspoon sesame oil

1 pound ground pork

1 red bell pepper, thinly sliced

8 corn tortillas

1 scallion, green and white parts, chopped

1 cup shredded cabbage (optional)

1. In a small mixing bowl, whisk together the garlic, orange zest, orange juice, sriracha, soy sauce, honey, cornstarch, and oil.

2. Heat a large skillet over medium-high heat.

3. Put the pork in the pan, and cook for about 5 minutes, or until browned. Drain off and discard any excess fat.

4. Add the bell pepper, and cook for 3 minutes, or until softened.

5. Pour in the sauce mixture, and stir constantly for 1 to 2 minutes, or until thickened. Remove from the heat.

6. Spoon the pork into the tortillas, and top with the scallion and cabbage (if using).

SUBSTITUTION TIP: If you don't have sriracha on hand, you can include a ½ teaspoon red pepper flakes to achieve the desired kick.

Per Serving: Calories: 391; Fat: 18g; Saturated Fat: 6g; Sodium: 279mg; Carbs: 34g; Fiber: 4g; Protein: 24g

Bánh Mì Pork Farro Bowls

30 MINUTES

Inspired by the classic Vietnamese bánh mì sandwich, these tasty bowls are guaranteed to fill your mouth with flavor. Plus, I wouldn't be surprised if quick-pickled vegetables, like the cucumber and carrot used in this dish, become your go-to topper for other sandwiches and salads.

Serves: 4   **Prep time:** 10 minutes   **Cook time:** 20 minutes

1 cup pearled farro, rinsed

2 cups water

½ cup vinegar

1 teaspoon salt

1 tablespoon sugar, plus 2 teaspoons

½ English cucumber

1 large carrot, peeled

1 pound ground pork

4 garlic cloves, minced

3 tablespoons reduced-sodium soy sauce

¼ teaspoon red pepper flakes

1 cup fresh cilantro

4 radishes, thinly sliced

1 jalapeño pepper, thinly sliced

Sriracha (optional)

2 teaspoons hemp seeds (optional)

1. In a 6-quart stockpot, combine the farro and water. Bring to a boil over high heat. Reduce the heat to medium-low, and simmer for 10 to 15 minutes, or until tender. Drain.

2. Meanwhile, whisk together the vinegar, salt, and 1 tablespoon of sugar in a bowl.

3. Using a vegetable peeler, thinly slice the cucumber and carrot. Add to the vinegar mixture, and cover.

4. Heat a large skillet over medium-high heat.

5. Put the pork in the pan, and cook for about 5 minutes, or until browned. Drain off and discard any excess fat.

6. Stir in the garlic, soy sauce, remaining 2 teaspoons of sugar, and the red pepper flakes. Cook for 1 minute, or until the sugar has dissolved. Remove from the heat.

7. Divide the farro among four bowls. Top with the pork, cucumbers, and carrots. Add the cilantro, radishes, and jalapeño pepper. Top with the sriracha (if using) and hemp seeds (if using) before serving.

SUBSTITUTION TIP: Toasted sesame seeds work just as well as hemp seeds here, so use those if they're easier to find.

Per Serving: Calories: 337; Fat: 7g; Saturated Fat: 2g; Sodium: 1115mg; Carbs: 39g; Fiber: 5g; Protein: 30g

Oven-Roasted Pork Chops with Apples and Walnuts

GLUTEN-FREE

There are fewer combinations as classically American as pork chops and apple-sauce. In this recipe, we put a heartwarming spin on tradition by seasoning apples and walnuts with cinnamon, nutmeg, thyme, and sage, before pairing them with the pork.

Serves: 4   **Prep time:** 10 minutes   **Cook time:** 25 minutes

2 medium apples, thinly sliced

2 tablespoons light brown sugar

1 teaspoon ground cinnamon

½ teaspoon dried thyme

¼ teaspoon dried sage

¼ teaspoon ground nutmeg

¼ cup chopped walnuts

4 boneless pork chops

Salt

Freshly ground black pepper

1. Preheat the oven to 400°F. Line a baking sheet with parchment paper or aluminum foil.

2. In a large bowl, combine the apples, sugar, cinnamon, thyme, sage, nutmeg, and walnuts. Spread onto the prepared baking sheet.

3. Put the pork chops on a clean cutting board, and cover with plastic wrap. Pound out the pork chops with a meat mallet or rolling pin until they're ¼-inch thick. Season both sides with salt and pepper, and place on top of the apples.

4. Transfer the baking sheet to the oven, and bake for 20 to 25 minutes, or until an instant-read thermometer inserted into the thickest part of the pork reaches an internal temperature of 145°F.

5. Transfer the pork to a serving dish, and top with the apples and walnuts before serving.

SERVING TIP: Serve these pork chops with a baked sweet potato topped with a dab of butter, cinnamon-spiced mashed potatoes, or garlicky green beans.

Per Serving: Calories: 348; Fat: 21g; Saturated Fat: 7g; Sodium: 241mg; Carbs: 21g; Fiber: 4g; Protein: 20g

Garlic-Herb Pork and Swiss Chard Pasta

30 MINUTES, ONE POT

Garlic lovers, this one's for you. Fresh herbs, such as parsley and basil, plus lemon and lots of garlic amplify the bright flavor of this pasta while still letting the Swiss chard shine. You'll love this leafy green for its mild taste and its supply of antioxidants, fiber, and vitamin A.

Serves: 4   **Prep time:** 10 minutes   **Cook time:** 15 minutes

1 pound whole-wheat farfalle

1 pound ground pork

4 garlic cloves, minced

1 teaspoon dried thyme

1 teaspoon salt

½ teaspoon freshly ground black pepper

1 large bunch green Swiss chard, stemmed and chopped

3 tablespoons fresh basil, chopped

3 tablespoons fresh parsley, chopped

2 tablespoons olive oil

1 teaspoon grated lemon zest

1 tablespoon freshly squeezed lemon juice

¼ cup grated Parmesan cheese

1. Cook the farfalle according to the package directions. Drain, and transfer to a bowl.

2. Heat the same pot over medium-high heat.

3. Put the pork in the pot, and cook for about 4 minutes, or until browned. Drain off and discard any excess fat.

4. Stir in the garlic, thyme, salt, and pepper. Cook for 30 seconds, or until fragrant.

5. Add the Swiss chard, and cook for about 2 minutes, or until wilted. Remove from the heat and transfer to the bowl with the farfalle.

6. Stir in the basil, parsley, oil, lemon zest, lemon juice, and cheese before serving.

SUBSTITUTION TIP: If you don't have fresh herbs on hand, use 1 tablespoon each of dried basil and dried parsley instead.

Per Serving: Calories: 653; Fat: 16g; Saturated Fat: 4g; Sodium: 643mg; Carbs: 79g; Fiber: 1g; Protein: 49g

Baked Tzatziki Pork Loin

GLUTEN-FREE

Tzatziki (tsah-SEE-key) is a traditional Greek dip made by combining yogurt with cucumber, garlic, and herbs. In this dish, smothering the pork loin in the yogurt mixture before roasting it in the oven locks in the juices and flavor—which is a fancy culinary way of saying, "It's out-of-this-world delicious."

Serves: 4   Prep time: 10 minutes, plus 10 minutes to chill   **Cook time:** 45 minutes

¾ cup plain Greek yogurt

2 tablespoons fresh dill, chopped

2 garlic cloves, minced

1½ tablespoons freshly squeezed lemon juice

1 tablespoon olive oil

½ teaspoon salt

½ English cucumber

1½ pounds pork loin, trimmed of excess fat

1. In a large bowl, combine the yogurt, dill, garlic, lemon juice, oil, and salt.

2. Using a box grater, grate the cucumber, and squeeze out the excess water with your hands before adding the cucumber to the yogurt. Stir until combined.

3. Add the pork, tossing to coat. Cover the bowl, and refrigerate for 10 minutes.

4. Preheat the oven to 400°F. Line a rimmed baking sheet with aluminum foil or parchment paper.

5. Transfer the pork to the baking sheet, and discard the marinade.

6. Transfer the baking sheet to the oven, and bake for 35 to 45 minutes, or until an instant-read thermometer inserted into the thickest part of the pork reaches an internal temperature of 145°F. Remove from the oven. Let rest for at least 5 minutes before slicing and serving.

SERVING TIP: This dish is perfectly complemented by garlicky mashed red potatoes or roasted potatoes tossed with olive oil, garlic, oregano, salt, and pepper.

Per Serving: Calories: 332; Fat: 19g; Saturated Fat: 7g; Sodium: 434mg; Carbs: 7g; Fiber: 1g; Protein: 35g

Beef, Mushroom, and Sweet Potato Cottage Pie

BUDGET

This humble dish, similar to shepherd's pie, is the epitome of comfort food. I like to add mushrooms to the ground beef because they contribute a certain richness while giving the meal a vitamin and mineral boost. Top the dish with a blanket of mashed sweet potatoes before baking, and you'll find yourself biting into a little slice of heaven.

Serves: 4   **Prep time:** 10 minutes   **Cook time:** 45 minutes

1 pound sweet potatoes, peeled and diced (about 3 medium potatoes)

1 teaspoon salt, divided, plus more as needed

1 teaspoon dried thyme

½ teaspoon dried sage

¼ teaspoon ground cinnamon

½ cup vegetable broth

1 pound lean ground beef

1 small yellow onion, chopped

10 ounces sliced button mushrooms

¼ teaspoon freshly ground black pepper, plus more as needed

1½ teaspoons Worcestershire sauce

2 cups frozen mixed vegetables, thawed

1. Preheat the oven to 400°F.
2. In a large stockpot, cover the sweet potatoes with water, and bring to a boil over high heat. Cook for 6 to 8 minutes, or until tender. Drain, and return to the pot.
3. Add ½ teaspoon of salt, the thyme, sage, cinnamon, and broth. Using a potato masher, mash until smooth.
4. Heat a large skillet over medium-high heat.
5. Put the ground beef in the pan, and cook for 4 to 5 minutes, or until browned. Drain off and discard any excess fat.
6. Add the onion and mushrooms to the pan, increase the heat to high, and cook for 5 to 6 minutes, or until the excess water from the mushrooms evaporates.
7. Add the remaining ½ teaspoon of salt, the pepper, and Worcestershire sauce, and cook for 1 minute, or until the flavors meld.
8. Transfer the beef mixture to an 8-inch-square baking dish, and top with the mixed vegetables. Cover evenly with the sweet potatoes. Season with salt and pepper, and cover with aluminum foil.

continued →

Beef, Mushroom, and Sweet Potato Cottage Pie *continued*

9. Transfer the baking dish to the oven, and bake for 20 minutes. Remove the foil, and bake for 5 minutes, or until the top is golden brown. Remove from the oven. Let rest for at least 5 minutes before serving.

DID YOU KNOW? Sweet potatoes are a rich source of vitamin A, a nutrient that supports eye health, immunity, and bone health.

Per Serving: Calories: 387; Fat: 11g; Saturated Fat: 5g; Sodium: 872mg; Carbs: 40g; Fiber: 9g; Protein: 31g

Steak, Kale, and Goat Cheese Quesadillas

5-INGREDIENT, 30 MINUTES, ONE POT

This quesadilla may be different from any you've had before—but in a good way. The tender steak pairs marvelously with the garlicky kale and creamy goat cheese, all of which is pressed into the perfect, crispy, tortilla package. Super family-friendly, these quesadillas are a great way to sneak in some vegetables.

Serves: 4   **Prep time:** 5 minutes   **Cook time:** 25 minutes

2 teaspoons canola oil

1 (8-ounce) strip steak, sliced thinly against the grain

1 large bunch kale, stemmed and chopped

2 garlic cloves, minced

⅓ cup water

4 (10-inch) whole-wheat tortillas

6 ounces goat cheese, softened

1. Heat a large skillet over high heat, and pour in the oil.

2. Add the steak, and cook for about 2 minutes per side, or until browned. Remove from the pan.

3. In the same pan, combine the kale, garlic, and water. Cook over high heat for about 5 minutes, or until wilted.

4. Add the steak back, stir to combine, and remove from the heat. Transfer to a plate. Wipe out the skillet with a damp paper towel.

5. Spread each tortilla with the goat cheese.

6. Spoon the steak mixture onto one half of each tortilla, and fold in half.

7. Heat the skillet over medium-high heat.

8. Add 1 prepared quesadilla. Cook for about 2 minutes per side, or until browned. Repeat the process with the remaining quesadillas, and serve.

Per Serving: Calories: 402; Fat: 19g; Saturated Fat: 6g; Sodium: 350mg; Carbs: 31g; Fiber: 5g; Protein: 27g

Beef-Stuffed Eggplant

BUDGET, GLUTEN-FREE

This go-to dinner dish plays with all the flavors of eggplant Parmesan, but it adds a boost of leafy greens and nixes the indulgent breading and deep-frying. What's even better: Each serving is already pre-portioned, meaning no more fighting over the last piece. Unless, of course, there are leftovers.

Serves: 4   **Prep time:** 10 minutes   **Cook time:** 40 minutes

2 medium eggplants

1 pound lean ground beef

1 small yellow onion, chopped

2 garlic cloves, minced

½ teaspoon dried oregano

½ teaspoon salt

¼ teaspoon freshly ground black pepper

1 cup marinara sauce

3 cups baby spinach

¼ cup grated Parmesan cheese

2 tablespoons fresh basil, chopped

1. Preheat the oven to 375°F. Line a rimmed baking sheet with aluminum foil.

2. Cut the eggplants in half lengthwise, and scoop out the flesh, leaving about a ½-inch border to keep the eggplant's shape intact. Roughly chop the scooped-out eggplant flesh.

3. Place the eggplant shells cut-side up on the baking sheet, and bake for 10 minutes, or until softened. Remove from the oven.

4. Meanwhile, heat a large skillet over high heat. Put the beef in the pan, and cook for about 5 minutes, or until browned. Drain off and discard any excess fat.

5. Stir in the chopped eggplant, onion, garlic, oregano, salt, and pepper. Cook for 3 minutes, or until fragrant.

6. Reduce the heat to low, and stir in the marinara sauce and spinach. Cook for about 2 minutes, or until the spinach has wilted.

7. Fill the eggplant shells with the beef mixture.

8. Top with the cheese, cover with foil, and bake for 25 minutes. Remove the foil, and bake for 5 minutes, or until cheese has browned. Top with the basil before serving.

DID YOU KNOW? Eggplant is a good source of fiber and also contains potassium and vitamin C.

Per Serving: Calories: 323; Fat: 12g; Saturated Fat: 6g; Sodium: 676mg; Carbs: 23g; Fiber: 9g; Protein: 30g

Thai Basil Beef–Stuffed Sweet Potatoes

30 MINUTES

Traditionally made with chicken, this beef version of a Thai dish strikes a harmonious balance between sweet and tangy, with a bit of a kick. By stuffing the ground beef into a sweet potato, we can give the dish a boost of fiber, vitamin A, and potassium—not to mention, temper the heat of the spicy serrano pepper.

Serves: 4   **Prep time:** 5 minutes   **Cook time:** 25 minutes

4 medium sweet potatoes

½ cup beef broth

3 tablespoons reduced-sodium soy sauce

1 tablespoon fish sauce

1 tablespoon vinegar

1 tablespoon honey

1 pound lean ground beef

3 garlic cloves, minced

1 serrano pepper, seeded and chopped

1 cup fresh basil leaves

1. Rinse the sweet potatoes, and pierce each with a fork. Place them on a microwave-safe plate, and microwave on high for 8 to 10 minutes, or until the flesh has softened. Split the sweet potatoes down the middle.

2. In a small bowl, whisk together the broth, soy sauce, fish sauce, vinegar, and honey.

3. Heat a large skillet over medium-high heat.

4. Put the beef in the pan, and cook for 4 to 5 minutes, or until browned.

5. Add the garlic and serrano pepper. Cook for 3 minutes, or until softened.

6. Pour the contents of the small bowl into the skillet, and increase the heat to high. Cook, stirring frequently, for 5 minutes, or until the sauce has thickened.

7. Add the basil, and cook for about 30 seconds, or until wilted. Remove from the heat, and spoon some beef into each sweet potato before serving.

SUBSTITUTION TIP: If you don't have fish sauce, Worcestershire sauce can be used instead.

Per Serving: Calories: 315; Fat: 8g; Saturated Fat: 3g; Sodium: 1038mg; Carbs: 33g; Fiber: 4g; Protein: 27g

Mongolian Beef and Bok Choy Quinoa Bowls

The key to this dish is all in the sauce. It's sticky, sweet, and salty, which is perfect for coating every bite of beef and bok choy with mouthwatering flavor. Bok choy adds some fiber and color, but any leafy green, like spinach or kale, can be used instead.

Serves: 4   **Prep time:** 10 minutes   **Cook time:** 25 minutes

2½ cups water, plus ¼ cup

2 cups quinoa, rinsed

3 garlic cloves, minced

1 tablespoon finely chopped fresh ginger

¼ cup reduced-sodium soy sauce

2 tablespoons maple syrup

2 tablespoons cornstarch

2 teaspoons canola oil

1 pound sirloin steak, sliced thinly against the grain

5 cups bok choy, stemmed and chopped

2 scallions, green and white parts, chopped

2 teaspoons hemp seeds (optional)

1. In a 4-quart stockpot, bring 2½ cups of water to a boil over high heat.

2. Add the quinoa, reduce the heat to low, and simmer for 10 to 15 minutes, or until tender.

3. In a small bowl, whisk together the garlic, ginger, soy sauce, remaining ¼ cup of water, the maple syrup, and cornstarch to make the sauce.

4. Heat a large skillet over medium-high heat, and pour in the oil.

5. Add the steak, and cook for 2 to 3 minutes per side, or until browned.

6. Add the bok choy and the sauce. Stir to coat, and cook, stirring frequently, for 2 to 3 minutes, or until the sauce has thickened and bok choy has wilted. Remove from the heat.

7. Divide the quinoa among four bowls, and top with the steak mixture. Sprinkle the scallions and hemp seeds (if using) on top.

SUBSTITUTION TIP: Sesame seeds are a good stand-in for hemp seeds.

Per Serving: Calories: 556; Fat: 12g; Saturated Fat: 1g; Sodium: 596mg; Carbs: 70g; Fiber: 7g; Protein: 40g

Spinach Caprese Beef Burgers

30 MINUTES, ONE POT

It's a Caprese salad. It's a burger. It's . . . both. Essentially, I've taken what I love about each to create this delicious hybrid. Combining the beef with balsamic vinegar, spinach, and mozzarella before topping the burgers with juicy tomato slices means that every bite exhibits the flavors of the beloved Italian salad.

Serves: 4   **Prep time:** 5 minutes   **Cook time:** 15 minutes

1 cup part-skim shredded mozzarella cheese, divided

1 cup baby spinach, finely chopped

1 pound lean ground beef

¼ cup basil, chopped

½ teaspoon salt

¼ teaspoon freshly ground black pepper

2 garlic cloves, minced

1 tablespoon balsamic vinegar

1 teaspoon canola oil

1 large tomato, sliced

4 hamburger buns

1. In a large mixing bowl, combine ½ cup of cheese, the spinach, beef, basil, salt, pepper, garlic, and vinegar.

2. Form the mixture into 4 patties, and create a small indent in the middle of each patty with your fingertips.

3. Heat a large skillet over medium-high heat, and pour in the oil.

4. Add the patties to the pan, and cook for 6 minutes on each side, or until cooked to your preferred doneness.

5. Top the patties with the remaining ½ cup of cheese. Remove from the heat, and cover the pan for 2 minutes, or until the cheese has melted.

6. Top each patty with sliced tomato before serving on hamburger buns.

DID YOU KNOW? Spinach is a natural source of antioxidants, fiber, and iron.

Per Serving: Calories: 397; Fat: 16g; Saturated Fat: 7g; Sodium: 645mg; Carbs: 26g; Fiber: 2g; Protein: 37g

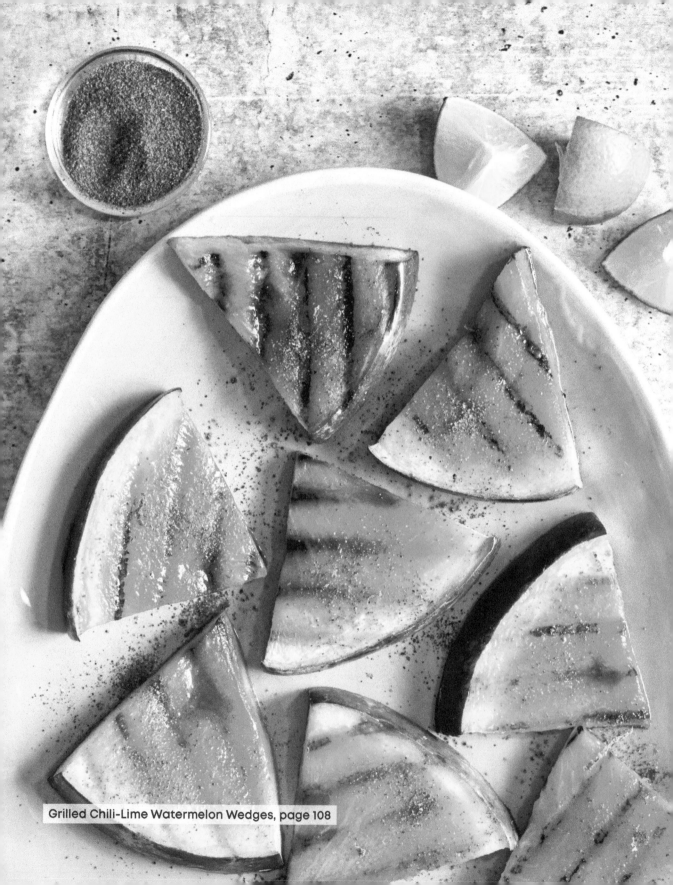

Grilled Chili-Lime Watermelon Wedges, page 108

8

Snacks and Desserts

Whether you need something to munch on or you're craving something sweet, the recipes in this chapter have you covered. You'll find a good mix of sweet and savory options incorporating fresh fruit and spices, as well as superfoods like walnuts, pumpkin seeds, and oats. The snacks, in particular, are a great way to sneak in a little extra nutrition between meals.

Super Seedy No-Bake Energy Bites

30 MINUTES, BUDGET, ONE POT, VEGAN

These energy bites are the perfect, popable snack to stock your refrigerator or freezer with for an on-the-go nutrition boost. The goji berries are a natural source of phytonutrients, which are plant compounds that have antioxidant and anti-inflammatory properties. The pumpkin seeds add a satisfying crunch and are full of magnesium, an essential mineral that is crucial for supporting both bone and heart health.

Serves: 12   **Prep time:** 15 minutes

2 cups rolled oats

¼ cup pumpkin seeds

¼ cup dried goji berries

2 tablespoons chia seeds

1 teaspoon ground cinnamon

½ cup unsweetened applesauce

¼ cup natural peanut butter

1 teaspoon vanilla extract

Olive oil, for your hands

1. In a large bowl, stir together the oats, pumpkin seeds, goji berries, chia seeds, and cinnamon.

2. Add the applesauce, peanut butter, and vanilla. Stir until combined.

3. Rub your hands with the oil (to prevent the mixture from sticking), and form the mixture into 12 balls.

4. Store the energy bites in an airtight container in the refrigerator for up to 4 days, or in the freezer for up to 2 weeks.

SUBSTITUTION TIP: If you don't have goji berries on hand, dried cranberries or dried cherries also work great.

Per Serving: Calories: 126; Fat: 6g; Saturated Fat: 1g; Sodium: 3mg; Carbs: 14g; Fiber: 3g; Protein: 5g

Savory Nori Popcorn

5-INGREDIENT, 30 MINUTES, BUDGET, ONE POT, VEGAN

This popcorn is a far cry from the overly salty, butter-drowned kind you'll find at the movie theater. The flavor here comes from tamari, a typically gluten-free soy sauce (always check product labeling), which adds a perfect, salty-rich flavor to complement the nori, a popular seaweed used in sushi making. Together, the two create a uniquely tasty popcorn topping.

Serves: 2   **Prep time:** 5 minutes   **Cook time:** 5 minutes

¼ cup popcorn kernels, divided

2 teaspoons canola oil

1 tablespoon reduced-sodium tamari

1 tablespoon finely chopped nori seaweed

½ teaspoon garlic powder (optional)

1. Heat a stockpot over medium heat.
2. Put 2 popcorn kernels and the oil in the pot, and cover.
3. Once both kernels have popped, add the remaining kernels, cover, and swirl the pot to coat the kernels with oil.
4. Continue cooking the kernels, swirling the pot frequently to prevent scorching.
5. Once the popping stops, turn off the heat, and transfer the popcorn to a large serving bowl.
6. Drizzle the popcorn with the tamari, and top with the nori and garlic powder (if using).

SUBSTITUTION TIP: If you don't have access to nori, replace it with 1 teaspoon of dried herbs, such as basil, oregano, or dill.

Per Serving: Calories: 165; Fat: 5g; Saturated Fat: 0g; Sodium: 312mg; Carbs: 23g; Fiber: 3g; Protein: 9g

Grilled Chili-Lime Watermelon Wedges

5-INGREDIENT, 30 MINUTES, BUDGET, GLUTEN-FREE, VEGAN

This may be the first time you'll add watermelon to a grill, but it certainly won't be the last. I guarantee you've never had watermelon quite like this; the combination of sweet, salty, and smoky will keep you and your guests coming back for more. If you don't have an outdoor grill, you can use a grill pan over medium-high heat instead.

Serves: 6 to 8   **Prep time:** 10 minutes   **Cook time:** 5 minutes

1 teaspoon chili powder

1 teaspoon grated lime zest

¼ teaspoon salt

¼ teaspoon sugar

1 small seedless watermelon, cut into wedges

Juice of 1 lime

1. Preheat the grill on high heat or a grill pan over medium-high heat.

2. In a small bowl, whisk together the chili powder, lime zest, salt, and sugar.

3. Place the watermelon directly on the grill, and cook for 2 minutes per side, or until grill marks appear. Transfer to a serving platter, and drizzle with the lime juice.

4. Top the watermelon with the chili powder mixture before serving.

SERVING TIP: The watermelon can be served warm, at room temperature, or refrigerated and served chilled.

Per Serving: Calories: 65; Fat: 0g; Saturated Fat: 0g; Sodium: 104mg; Carbs: 16g; Fiber: 1g; Protein: 1g

Savory Chickpea, Feta, and Arugula Yogurt Bowl

30 MINUTES, BUDGET, GLUTEN-FREE, ONE POT, VEGETARIAN

We often think of the sweet, fruity side of yogurt bowls, but savory versions like this one deserve a try as well. Here, the thick and creamy texture of the Greek yogurt goes hand in hand with the peppery arugula and the tang of the feta cheese. Not only is this snack full of hunger-crushing protein and fiber—the olive oil and hemp seeds each provide a dose of healthy fats to help absorb the recipe's fat-soluble vitamins.

Serves: 1   **Prep time:** 5 minutes

1 cup plain, low-fat
  Greek yogurt

⅓ cup chickpeas

½ cup arugula,
  coarsely chopped

2 tablespoons crumbled
  feta cheese

1 teaspoon hemp seeds

1 teaspoon olive oil

1 teaspoon
  balsamic vinegar

Salt

Freshly ground
  black pepper

1. Spoon the yogurt into a small bowl.
2. Top with the chickpeas, arugula, cheese, and hemp seeds.
3. Drizzle with the oil and balsamic vinegar, and season with salt and pepper.

SUBSTITUTION TIP: Chopped walnuts or almonds are a simple and delicious substitute for hemp seeds.

Per Serving: Calories: 350; Fat: 13g; Saturated Fat: 4g; Sodium: 386mg; Carbs: 26g; Fiber: 4g; Protein: 33g

Ginger Matcha "Nice" Cream

5-INGREDIENT, 30 MINUTES, BUDGET, GLUTEN-FREE, ONE POT, VEGAN

Few things rival the yumminess of five-minute homemade ice cream—except perhaps *healthy* five-minute homemade ice cream. In this version, matcha, a concentrated green tea powder, adds a dose of antioxidants and an earthy flavor that stands up nicely to the spice of fresh ginger. The base of frozen bananas gives this ice cream its creamy texture and sweetness without the need for added sugars.

Serves: 2   Prep time: 5 minutes

4 ripe bananas, sliced and frozen

2 tablespoons unsweetened vanilla almond milk

1 tablespoon matcha powder

1 teaspoon grated fresh ginger

1. In a blender or food processor, combine the bananas, almond milk, matcha, and ginger.

2. Blend on high for 1 minute, or until smooth.

3. Transfer the mixture to a bowl and serve as is, or transfer it to a container and freeze for 1 hour for a firmer texture.

SUBSTITUTION TIP: No fresh ginger on hand? No problem. Use ¼ teaspoon of ground ginger instead.

Per Serving: Calories: 230; Fat: 1g; Saturated Fat: 0g; Sodium: 14mg; Carbs: 59g; Fiber: 7g; Protein: 3g

Trail Mix Cookies

30 MINUTES, BUDGET, VEGAN

If you've been looking for a nutritious way to satisfy your afternoon sweet tooth, bake a batch of these chunky, just-sweet-enough cookies. Besides being delicious, they don't contain any added sweeteners and are full of nutrient-rich nuts, seeds, and fiber-filled oats to keep you going for the rest of the day.

Serves: 12   **Prep time:** 10 minutes   **Cook time:** 15 minutes

2½ cups rolled oats

¼ cup chopped walnuts

¼ cup pumpkin seeds

¼ cup dried goji berries

2 tablespoons ground flaxseed (optional)

2 teaspoons ground cinnamon

½ teaspoon baking powder

2 very ripe bananas

2 teaspoons vanilla extract

¼ cup natural peanut butter

1. Preheat the oven to 350°F. Line a baking sheet with parchment paper.
2. In a large bowl, stir together the oats, walnuts, pumpkin seeds, goji berries, flaxseed (if using), cinnamon, and baking powder.
3. In a small bowl, mash the bananas until smooth. Stir in the vanilla and peanut butter.
4. To make the cookie dough, add the banana mixture to the oats, and stir to combine.
5. Roll the cookie dough into 12 golf ball–size portions. Place on the prepared baking sheet, and flatten slightly with the back of a spoon or your fingertips.
6. Transfer the baking sheet to the oven, and bake for 12 to 15 minutes, or until firm. Remove from the oven.
7. Let the cookies cool on the baking sheet for 5 minutes before transferring to a wire rack to cool completely. Store leftovers in the refrigerator for up to 4 days.

SUBSTITUTION TIP: No goji berries? Dried cranberries or dried cherries will give you the same hint of sweetness.

Per Serving: Calories: 113; Fat: 6g; Saturated Fat: 1g; Sodium: 2mg; Carbs: 12g; Fiber: 2g; Protein: 4g

Raspberry-Coconut Oatmeal Bars

BUDGET, VEGAN

Get ready to go coco-nuts for these fantastic bars. The sweet, tart flavor of fresh raspberries with a touch of lemon mingles with the toasted oats, coconut, and cinnamon to form a downright irresistible snack. You might want to store these hidden in the back of the refrigerator—if they even make it there, that is.

Serves: 9   **Prep time:** 10 minutes   **Cook time:** 40 minutes

1 cup rolled oats

½ cup all-purpose flour

½ cup shredded coconut

⅓ cup light brown
  sugar, plus
  1 tablespoon, packed

½ teaspoon
  baking powder

¼ teaspoon salt

¼ teaspoon
  ground cinnamon

⅓ cup canola oil

2 cups fresh or frozen and
  thawed raspberries

1 teaspoon grated
  lemon zest

1 tablespoon freshly
  squeezed lemon juice

1. Preheat the oven to 375°F. Line an 8-inch-square baking dish with parchment paper.

2. In a large bowl, whisk together the oats, flour, coconut, ⅓ cup of brown sugar, baking powder, salt, and cinnamon.

3. Stir in the oil until the mixture is crumbly.

4. Reserve 1 cup of the oat mixture, and pour the rest into the prepared baking dish. Using your fingertips or a spatula, press the oat mixture firmly into the pan, making sure to cover the bottom.

5. In the same bowl, combine the raspberries, the remaining 1 tablespoon of brown sugar, the lemon zest, and lemon juice. Using a spoon or spatula, mash the berries, and spread the berry mixture evenly over the crust in the baking dish.

6. Sprinkle the reserved oat mixture over the berry mixture, and press down firmly.

7. Transfer the baking dish to the oven, and bake for 35 to 40 minutes, or until golden brown. Remove from the oven.

8. Once the baking dish is cool to the touch, transfer it to the refrigerator and let the bars cool completely before cutting into 9 pieces. Store the bars in the refrigerator for a firmer texture.

SUBSTITUTION TIP: These bars are delicious when made with any berries you have on hand, such as blueberries, strawberries, or blackberries, or a mix of all three.

Per Serving: Calories: 182; Fat: 10g; Saturated Fat: 2g; Sodium: 70mg; Carbs: 21g; Fiber: 3g; Protein: 2g

Chocolate, Strawberry, and Avocado Mousse

5-INGREDIENT, 30 MINUTES, GLUTEN-FREE, ONE POT, VEGAN

If you love chocolate-covered strawberries, then you'll want to give this decadently healthy dessert a try. A base of creamy avocado makes this mousse taste indulgent, but it actually contains healthy fats, fiber, and antioxidants. In this dessert, cacao powder, a less processed cocoa powder with a rich chocolate flavor, is sweetened with preserves and fresh strawberries.

Serves: 4   **Prep time:** 5 minutes

2 ripe avocados, pitted and peeled

½ cup unsweetened, vanilla almond milk

6 tablespoons cacao powder

¼ cup strawberry preserves

1 tablespoon maple syrup (optional)

½ cup fresh strawberries, chopped

1. In a blender, combine the avocados, almond milk, cacao powder, and strawberry preserves. Blend on high for 1 minute, or until smooth. Transfer to a serving bowl.

2. Stir in the maple syrup (if using).

3. Add the strawberries, and stir to combine before serving.

SUBSTITUTION TIP: If you don't have cacao powder on hand, regular cocoa powder will work just fine.

Per Serving: Calories: 306; Fat: 20g; Saturated Fat: 6g; Sodium: 30mg; Carbs: 43g; Fiber: 15g; Protein: 8g

Peanut Butter–Stuffed Baked Apples

BUDGET, VEGAN

You've never truly experienced the greatness of baked apples if you haven't had them stuffed with peanut butter. These beauties have a touch of brown sugar and are baked until they're warm and bubbly. If you happen to have a peanut allergy, subbing in almond butter or sunflower seed butter will produce an equally drool-worthy result.

Serves: 4   **Prep time:** 10 minutes   **Cook time:** 30 minutes

4 medium apples

¼ cup natural chunky peanut butter

1 teaspoon cinnamon, plus ½ teaspoon

1 teaspoon vanilla extract

¼ cup rolled oats

2 tablespoons light brown sugar

1 tablespoon canola oil

1. Preheat the oven to 400°F. Line an 8-inch-square baking dish with aluminum foil.

2. Scoop out the cores and seeds from the apples, leaving the bottoms intact. Place the apples standing up in the prepared baking dish.

3. In a small bowl, mix together the peanut butter, 1 teaspoon of cinnamon, and the vanilla. Drop the mixture by the spoonful into the prepared apples.

4. In the same bowl, mix together the oats, sugar, remaining ½ teaspoon of cinnamon, and the oil. Press the mixture firmly onto the top of each apple.

5. Transfer the baking dish to the oven, and bake for 20 to 30 minutes, or until the apples are tender. Remove from the oven. Serve immediately.

SERVING TIP: Take these apples up a notch by serving them accompanied by a scoop of fresh whipped cream or vanilla ice cream.

Per Serving: Calories: 283; Fat: 12g; Saturated Fat: 1g; Sodium: 4mg; Carbs: 43g; Fiber: 8g; Protein: 6g

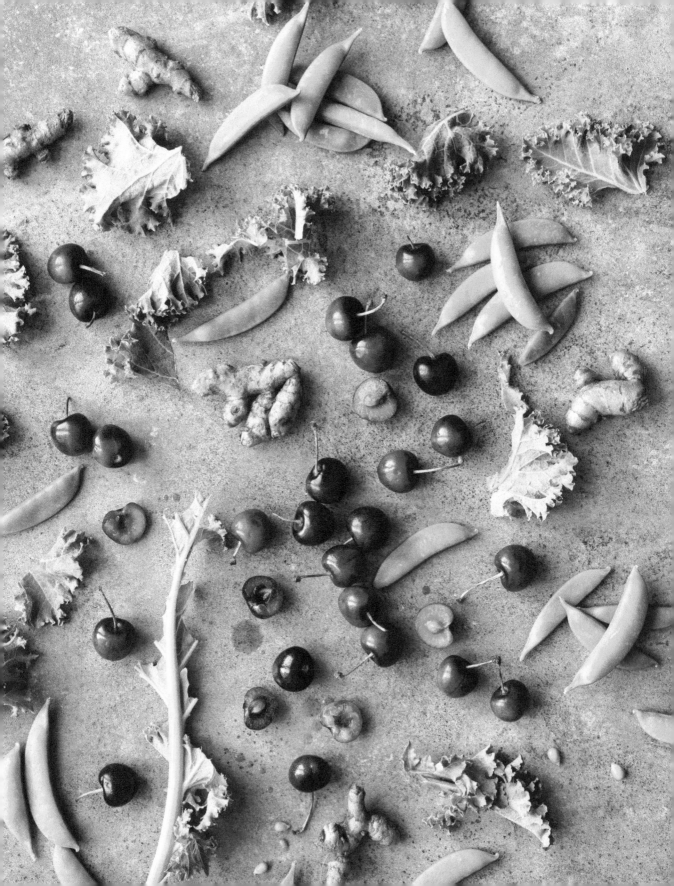

Measurement Conversions

VOLUME EQUIVALENTS (LIQUID)

US STANDARD	US STANDARD (OUNCES)	METRIC (APPROXIMATE)
2 tablespoons	1 fl. oz.	30 mL
¼ cup	2 fl. oz.	60 mL
½ cup	4 fl. oz.	120 mL
1 cup	8 fl. oz.	240 mL
1½ cups	12 fl. oz.	355 mL
2 cups or 1 pint	16 fl. oz.	475 mL
4 cups or 1 quart	32 fl. oz.	1 L
1 gallon	128 fl. oz.	4 L

OVEN TEMPERATURES

FAHRENHEIT	CELSIUS (APPROXIMATE)
250°F	120°C
300°F	150°C
325°F	165°C
350°F	180°C
375°F	190°C
400°F	200°C
425°F	220°C
450°F	230°C

VOLUME EQUIVALENTS (DRY)

US STANDARD	METRIC (APPROXIMATE)
⅛ teaspoon	0.5 mL
¼ teaspoon	1 mL
½ teaspoon	2 mL
¾ teaspoon	4 mL
1 teaspoon	5 mL
1 tablespoon	15 mL
¼ cup	59 mL
⅓ cup	79 mL
½ cup	118 mL
⅔ cup	156 mL
¾ cup	177 mL
1 cup	235 mL
2 cups or 1 pint	475 mL
3 cups	700 mL
4 cups or 1 quart	1 L

WEIGHT EQUIVALENTS

US STANDARD	METRIC (APPROXIMATE)
½ ounce	15 g
1 ounce	30 g
2 ounces	60 g
4 ounces	115 g
8 ounces	225 g
12 ounces	340 g
16 ounces or 1 pound	455 g

Resources

- The Dietary Guidelines for Americans (https://health.gov/dietaryguide lines/): Here you'll find the most current evidence-based dietary recommendations from the United States Department of Agriculture.

- EatRight.org: The official website of the Academy of Nutrition and Dietetics, this site is a resource for evidence-based nutrition research and recommendations.

- *The Flavor Bible: The Essential Guide to Culinary Creativity, Based on the Wisdom of America's Most Imaginative Chefs* by Karen Page and Andrew Dornenburg: A valuable book for discovering flavor pairings and how to use a variety of herbs and spices.

- The National Institutes of Health Dietary Supplement Fact Sheets (https:// ods.od.nih.gov/factsheets/list-all/): This site offers evidence-based information on dietary supplements, vitamins, and minerals.

- USDA FoodData Central (https://fdc.nal.usda.gov/): This is a reliable source of nutrition information for food and food items.

References

Chen, Fan, Mengxi Du, Jeffrey B. Blumberg, Kenneth Kwan Ho Chui, Mengyuan Ruan, Gail Rogers, Zhilei Shan, Luxian Zeng, and Fang Fang Zhang. "Association Among Dietary Supplement Use, Nutrient Intake, and Mortality Among U.S. Adults." *Annals of Internal Medicine* 170, no. 9 (2019): 604–13. doi:10.7326/m18-2478.

Harvard T.H. Chan School of Public Health. "Superfoods or Superhype?" *The Nutrition Source*. July 1, 2019. https://www.hsph.harvard.edu/nutritionsource /superfoods/.

Royston, Kendra J., and Trygve O. Tollefsbol. "The Epigenetic Impact of Cruciferous Vegetables on Cancer Prevention." *Current Pharmacology Reports* 1, no. 1 (February 2015): 46–51. doi:10.1007/s40495-014-0003-9.

U.S. Department of Agriculture. "Food Data Central." Agricultural Research Service. https://fdc.nal.usda.gov/.

U.S. Department of Health and Human Services. "Dietary Supplement Fact Sheets." NIH Office of Dietary Supplements. https://ods.od.nih.gov/factsheets/list-all/.

Recipe Index

A

Arugula and Goat Cheese–Stuffed Chicken Breasts, 82

Autumn Lentil Farro Bowls, 62

B

Baked Radishes with Balsamic Vinegar, 55

Baked Tzatziki Pork Loin, 96

Bánh Mì Pork Farro Bowls, 93

Beef, Mushroom, and Sweet Potato Cottage Pie, 97–98

Beef-Stuffed Eggplant, 100

Blackened Salmon Taco Salad, 53

C

Chocolate, Strawberry, and Avocado Mousse, 114

Chocolate-Covered Cherry Smoothie, 28

Citrus-Strawberry Smoothie, 21

Coconut-Lime Shrimp Tacos, 79

Cold Brew Mocha Smoothie, 26

Creamy Avocado and Split Pea Soup, 44

Creamy Butternut Squash and Kale Linguine, 60

Creamy Pineapple-Cilantro Smoothie, 23

Crispy Pecan-Baked Chicken, 83

Crunchy Bok Choy Slaw, 52

Curry Vegetable Peanut Stew, 45

G

Garlic-Herb Pork and Swiss Chard Pasta, 95

Ginger Matcha "Nice" Cream, 110

Ginger-Sesame Tuna Wraps, 77

Golden Milk Oatmeal with Toasted Pecans, 33

Greek Turkey and Barley–Stuffed Peppers, 86–87

Gremolata-Stuffed Tilapia, 76

Grilled Chicken with Pineapple-Avocado Salsa, 81

Grilled Chili-Lime Watermelon Wedges, 108

Grilled Romaine Chickpea Caesar Salad, 51

L

Lemony Blueberry-Basil Smoothie, 22

Lentil-Walnut Tacos, 72

M

Maple-Dijon Sautéed Kale, 54

Miso Soup with Bok Choy and Tofu, 42

Mongolian Beef and Bok Choy Quinoa Bowls, 102

Mushroom, Kale, and Farro Risotto, 61

O

One-Pot Three-Bean Chili, 46

One-Pot Turkey Pasta Primavera, 89

Orange and Sriracha Pork Tacos, 92

Oven-Roasted Pork Chops with Apples and Walnuts, 94

P

Pan-Seared Scallops over Lemon-Basil Farro, 80

Peanut Butter–Stuffed Baked Apples, 115

Pineapple Curry Turkey Burgers, 88

Pistachio-Crusted Salmon, 78

Pomegranate-Broccoli Salad, 49

Pumpkin-Spiced Buckwheat Pancakes, 34

Q

Quinoa Breakfast Power Bowls, 36–37

R

Raspberry-Coconut Oatmeal Bars, 112–113

Refreshing Watermelon-Mint Smoothie, 20

Ricotta, Blackberry, and Arugula Flatbreads, 64

Roasted Red Pepper and White Bean Shakshuka, 71

Roasted Root Vegetable Hash, 35

S

Savory Chickpea, Feta, and Arugula Yogurt Bowl, 109

Savory Nori Popcorn, 107

Shredded Pesto Chicken Quinoa Bowls, 84–85

Spicy Black Bean and Avocado Overnight Oats, 32

Spicy Peanut-Tofu Collard Wraps, 66–67

Spicy Sesame Chicken Noodle Soup, 43

Spinach and Artichoke Frittata, 38

Spinach and Feta Chickpea Burgers, 65

Spinach Caprese Beef Burgers, 103

Spinach, Walnut, and Goat Cheese–Stuffed Portobello Mushrooms, 63

Steak, Kale, and Goat Cheese Quesadillas, 99

Summer Vegetable Lasagna with Tofu Ricotta, 58–59

Super Green Smoothie Bowl, 24

Super Seedy No-Bake Energy Bites, 106

Sweet Corn Clam Chowder, 48

Sweet Potato and Black Bean Burritos, 70

Sweet Potato Pie Smoothie, 29

T

Tempeh Taco Bowls, 73

Thai Basil Beef–Stuffed Sweet Potatoes, 101

Thai Sweet Potato Salad, 50

Tofu Spaghetti Squash Pad Thai, 68–69

Trail Mix Cookies, 111

Triple Berry Kefir Smoothie, 27

Turkey-Pumpkin Chili, 47

V

Vanilla Matcha Latte Smoothie, 25

Index

A

Açai berries, 8

Triple Berry Kefir
Smoothie, 27

Almond milk

Chocolate, Strawberry,
and Avocado
Mousse, 114

Chocolate-Covered
Cherry Smoothie, 28

Cold Brew Mocha
Smoothie, 26

Creamy
Pineapple-Cilantro
Smoothie, 23

Ginger Matcha "Nice"
Cream, 110

Golden Milk Oatmeal with
Toasted Pecans, 33

Lemony Blueberry-Basil
Smoothie, 22

Pumpkin-Spiced
Buckwheat
Pancakes, 34

Super Green Smoothie
Bowl, 24

Sweet Potato Pie
Smoothie, 29

Vanilla Matcha Latte
Smoothie, 25

Almonds, 4

Crunchy Bok Choy
Slaw, 52

Apples, 3

Autumn Lentil Farro
Bowls, 62

Oven-Roasted Pork
Chops with Apples and
Walnuts, 94

Peanut Butter-Stuffed
Baked Apples, 115

Pomegranate-Broccoli
Salad, 49

Artichoke hearts

Spinach and Artichoke
Frittata, 38

Arugula, 6

Arugula and Goat
Cheese-Stuffed
Chicken Breasts, 82

Ricotta, Blackberry, and
Arugula Flatbreads, 64

Savory Chickpea, Feta,
and Arugula Yogurt
Bowl, 109

Avocados, 3

Blackened Salmon Taco
Salad, 53

Chocolate, Strawberry,
and Avocado
Mousse, 114

Creamy Avocado and
Split Pea Soup, 44

Creamy
Pineapple-Cilantro
Smoothie, 23

Grilled Chicken with
Pineapple-Avocado
Salsa, 81

Quinoa Breakfast Power
Bowls, 36–37

Spicy Black Bean and
Avocado Overnight
Oats, 32

Tempeh Taco Bowls, 73

B

Bananas, 13

Cold Brew Mocha
Smoothie, 26

Ginger Matcha "Nice"
Cream, 110

Sweet Potato Pie
Smoothie, 29

Trail Mix Cookies, 111

Vanilla Matcha Latte
Smoothie, 25

Barley, 5

Greek Turkey and
Barley-Stuffed
Peppers, 86–87

Barramundi, 10

Basil

Beef-Stuffed
Eggplant, 100

Garlic-Herb Pork and
Swiss Chard Pasta, 95

Lemony Blueberry-Basil
Smoothie, 22

Pan-Seared Scallops over
Lemon-Basil Farro, 80

Ricotta, Blackberry, and
Arugula Flatbreads, 64

Roasted Red Pepper
and White Bean
Shakshuka, 71

Spinach Caprese Beef
Burgers, 103

Thai Basil Beef-Stuffed
Sweet Potatoes, 101

Beans. See specific

Beef

Beef, Mushroom, and
Sweet Potato Cottage
Pie, 97–98

Beef-Stuffed
Eggplant, 100

Mongolian Beef and
Bok Choy Quinoa
Bowls, 102

Spinach Caprese Beef
Burgers, 103

Steak, Kale, and Goat
Cheese Quesadillas, 99
Thai Basil Beef–Stuffed
Sweet Potatoes, 101
Beets, 9
Roasted Root Vegetable
Hash, 35
Bell peppers
Curry Vegetable Peanut
Stew, 45
Greek Turkey and Barley–
Stuffed Peppers, 86–87
One-Pot Three-Bean
Chili, 46
One-Pot Turkey Pasta
Primavera, 89
Orange and Sriracha Pork
Tacos, 92
Roasted Red Pepper
and White Bean
Shakshuka, 71
Spicy Sesame Chicken
Noodle Soup, 43
Summer Vegetable
Lasagna with Tofu
Ricotta, 58–59
Turkey-Pumpkin Chili, 47
Berries. *See specific*
Bibb lettuce
Ginger-Sesame Tuna
Wraps, 77
Black beans, 9
Blackened Salmon Taco
Salad, 53
One-Pot Three-Bean
Chili, 46
Spicy Black Bean and
Avocado Overnight
Oats, 32
Sweet Potato and Black
Bean Burritos, 70
Blackberries, 3
Ricotta, Blackberry, and
Arugula Flatbreads, 64

Blueberries, 3
Lemony Blueberry-Basil
Smoothie, 22
Super Green Smoothie
Bowl, 24
Triple Berry Kefir
Smoothie, 27
Bok choy, 6
Crunchy Bok Choy
Slaw, 52
Miso Soup with Bok Choy
and Tofu, 42
Mongolian Beef and
Bok Choy Quinoa
Bowls, 102
Bowls
Autumn Lentil Farro
Bowls, 62
Bánh Mì Pork Farro
Bowls, 93
Mongolian Beef and
Bok Choy Quinoa
Bowls, 102
Quinoa Breakfast Power
Bowls, 36–37
Shredded Pesto Chicken
Quinoa Bowls, 84–85
Super Green Smoothie
Bowl, 24
Tempeh Taco Bowls, 73
Brazil nuts, 4
Broccoli, 6
One-Pot Turkey Pasta
Primavera, 89
Pomegranate-Broccoli
Salad, 49
Brown rice, 13
Buckwheat, 5
Budget
Autumn Lentil Farro
Bowls, 62
Baked Radishes with
Balsamic Vinegar, 55

Beef, Mushroom, and
Sweet Potato Cottage
Pie, 97–98
Beef-Stuffed
Eggplant, 100
Creamy Avocado and
Split Pea Soup, 44
Creamy Butternut
Squash and Kale
Linguine, 60
Ginger Matcha "Nice"
Cream, 110
Ginger-Sesame Tuna
Wraps, 77
Golden Milk Oatmeal
with Toasted
Pecans, 33
Greek Turkey and
Barley–Stuffed
Peppers, 86–87
Gremolata-Stuffed
Tilapia, 76
Grilled Chili-Lime
Watermelon
Wedges, 108
Grilled Romaine
Chickpea Caesar
Salad, 51
Lentil-Walnut Tacos, 72
Mushroom, Kale, and
Farro Risotto, 61
One-Pot Three-Bean
Chili, 46
Orange and Sriracha Pork
Tacos, 92
Peanut Butter–Stuffed
Baked Apples, 115
Pineapple Curry Turkey
Burgers, 88
Raspberry-Coconut
Oatmeal Bars, 112–113
Ricotta, Blackberry,
and Arugula
Flatbreads, 64

Budget *(Continued)*

Roasted Red Pepper and White Bean Shakshuka, 71

Roasted Root Vegetable Hash, 35

Savory Chickpea, Feta, and Arugula Yogurt Bowl, 109

Savory Nori Popcorn, 107

Spicy Black Bean and Avocado Overnight Oats, 32

Spicy Peanut-Tofu Collard Wraps, 66–67

Spinach and Artichoke Frittata, 38

Spinach and Feta Chickpea Burgers, 65

Spinach, Walnut, and Goat Cheese–Stuffed Portobello Mushrooms, 63

Summer Vegetable Lasagna with Tofu Ricotta, 58–59

Super Seedy No-Bake Energy Bites, 106

Sweet Corn Clam Chowder, 48

Sweet Potato and Black Bean Burritos, 70

Tempeh Taco Bowls, 73

Tofu Spaghetti Squash Pad Thai, 68–69

Trail Mix Cookies, 111

Burgers

Pineapple Curry Turkey Burgers, 88

Spinach and Feta Chickpea Burgers, 65

Spinach Caprese Beef Burgers, 103

C

Cabbage. *See also* **Coleslaw; Kimchi; Sauerkraut**

Coconut-Lime Shrimp Tacos, 79

Orange and Sriracha Pork Tacos, 92

Calcium, 7

Cannellini beans, 9

Cantaloupe, 13

Carrots, 9

Bánh Mì Pork Farro Bowls, 93

Creamy Avocado and Split Pea Soup, 44

Crunchy Bok Choy Slaw, 52

Curry Vegetable Peanut Stew, 45

One-Pot Three-Bean Chili, 46

Roasted Root Vegetable Hash, 35

Spicy Peanut-Tofu Collard Wraps, 66–67

Spicy Sesame Chicken Noodle Soup, 43

Cauliflower

Chocolate-Covered Cherry Smoothie, 28

Celery, 13

Creamy Avocado and Split Pea Soup, 44

Sweet Corn Clam Chowder, 48

Cheddar cheese

Sweet Potato and Black Bean Burritos, 70

Cheese. *See specific*

Cherries, 4

Chocolate-Covered Cherry Smoothie, 28

Chia seeds, 8

Cold Brew Mocha Smoothie, 26

Spicy Black Bean and Avocado Overnight Oats, 32

Super Green Smoothie Bowl, 24

Super Seedy No-Bake Energy Bites, 106

Vanilla Matcha Latte Smoothie, 25

Chicken

Arugula and Goat Cheese–Stuffed Chicken Breasts, 82

Crispy Pecan-Baked Chicken, 83

Grilled Chicken with Pineapple-Avocado Salsa, 81

Shredded Pesto Chicken Quinoa Bowls, 84–85

Spicy Sesame Chicken Noodle Soup, 43

Chickpeas, 9–10

Greek Turkey and Barley-Stuffed Peppers, 86–87

Grilled Romaine Chickpea Caesar Salad, 51

Savory Chickpea, Feta, and Arugula Yogurt Bowl, 109

Spinach and Feta Chickpea Burgers, 65

Chocolate

Chocolate, Strawberry, and Avocado Mousse, 114

Chocolate-Covered Cherry Smoothie, 28

Cold Brew Mocha Smoothie, 26

Cilantro
Bánh Mì Pork Farro
Bowls, 93
Creamy
Pineapple-Cilantro
Smoothie, 23
Grilled Chicken with
Pineapple-Avocado
Salsa, 81
Sweet Potato and Black
Bean Burritos, 70
Tempeh Taco Bowls, 73

Clams, 10
Sweet Corn Clam
Chowder, 48

Coconut
Coconut-Lime Shrimp
Tacos, 79
Raspberry-Coconut
Oatmeal Bars, 112–113
Super Green Smoothie
Bowl, 24

Coconut milk
Coconut-Lime Shrimp
Tacos, 79

Coleslaw
Spicy Peanut-Tofu Collard
Wraps, 66–67

Collard greens, 6
Spicy Peanut-Tofu Collard
Wraps, 66–67

Corn
Blackened Salmon Taco
Salad, 53
One-Pot Three-Bean
Chili, 46
Sweet Corn Clam
Chowder, 48
Sweet Potato and Black
Bean Burritos, 70
Tempeh Taco Bowls, 73
Turkey-Pumpkin Chili, 47

Cranberries, dried
Autumn Lentil Farro
Bowls, 62

Cucumbers, 13
Baked Tzatziki Pork
Loin, 96
Bánh Mì Pork Farro
Bowls, 93
Spicy Peanut-Tofu Collard
Wraps, 66–67

D

Desserts
Chocolate, Strawberry,
and Avocado
Mousse, 114
Ginger Matcha "Nice"
Cream, 110
Peanut Butter-Stuffed
Baked Apples, 115
Raspberry-Coconut
Oatmeal Bars, 112–113
Trail Mix Cookies, 111

Dill
Baked Tzatziki Pork
Loin, 96
Pistachio-Crusted
Salmon, 78

E

Edamame
Curry Vegetable Peanut
Stew, 45

Eggplants
Beef-Stuffed
Eggplant, 100
Summer Vegetable
Lasagna with Tofu
Ricotta, 58–59

Eggs, 11
Quinoa Breakfast Power
Bowls, 36–37

Roasted Red Pepper
and White Bean
Shakshuka, 71
Spinach and Artichoke
Frittata, 38
Tofu Spaghetti Squash
Pad Thai, 68–69

Equipment, 15–16

F

Farro, 5
Autumn Lentil Farro
Bowls, 62
Bánh Mì Pork Farro
Bowls, 93
Mushroom, Kale, and
Farro Risotto, 61
Pan-Seared Scallops
over Lemon-Basil
Farro, 80

Fats, 11

Feta cheese
Greek Turkey and
Barley-Stuffed
Peppers, 86–87
Roasted Red Pepper
and White Bean
Shakshuka, 71
Savory Chickpea, Feta,
and Arugula Yogurt
Bowl, 109
Spinach and Feta
Chickpea Burgers, 65

Fish, 10–11. *See also specific*

5-ingredient
Chocolate-Covered
Cherry Smoothie, 28
Citrus-Strawberry
Smoothie, 21
Ginger Matcha "Nice"
Cream, 110
Pistachio-Crusted
Salmon, 78

5-ingredient *(Continued)*
    Refreshing Watermelon-
        Mint Smoothie, 20
    Savory Nori Popcorn, 107
    Triple Berry Kefir
        Smoothie, 27
Flaxseed, 8
    Trail Mix Cookies, 111
Freezer staples, 12
Fruits, 3–4. *See also specific*

G
Garlic, 13
Ginger, 11
    Ginger Matcha "Nice"
        Cream, 110
    Ginger-Sesame Tuna
        Wraps, 77
    Mongolian Beef and
        Bok Choy Quinoa
        Bowls, 102
    Pineapple Curry Turkey
        Burgers, 88
    Spicy Peanut-Tofu Collard
        Wraps, 66–67
    Spicy Sesame Chicken
        Noodle Soup, 43
    Thai Sweet Potato
        Salad, 50
Gluten-free
    Arugula and Goat
        Cheese–Stuffed
        Chicken Breasts, 82
    Baked Radishes with
        Balsamic Vinegar, 55
    Baked Tzatziki Pork
        Loin, 96
    Beef-Stuffed
        Eggplant, 100
    Blackened Salmon Taco
        Salad, 53
    Chocolate, Strawberry,
        and Avocado
        Mousse, 114

Chocolate-Covered
    Cherry Smoothie, 28
Citrus-Strawberry
    Smoothie, 21
Coconut-Lime Shrimp
    Tacos, 79
Cold Brew Mocha
    Smoothie, 26
Creamy Avocado and
    Split Pea Soup, 44
Creamy
    Pineapple-Cilantro
    Smoothie, 23
Crispy Pecan-Baked
    Chicken, 83
Curry Vegetable Peanut
    Stew, 45
Ginger Matcha "Nice"
    Cream, 110
Ginger-Sesame Tuna
    Wraps, 77
Gremolata-Stuffed
    Tilapia, 76
Grilled Chicken with
    Pineapple-Avocado
    Salsa, 81
Grilled Chili-Lime
    Watermelon
    Wedges, 108
Lemony Blueberry-Basil
    Smoothie, 22
Lentil-Walnut Tacos, 72
Maple-Dijon Sautéed
    Kale, 54
One-Pot Three-Bean
    Chili, 46
Oven-Roasted Pork
    Chops with Apples and
    Walnuts, 94
Pineapple Curry Turkey
    Burgers, 88
Pistachio-Crusted
    Salmon, 78
Pomegranate-Broccoli
    Salad, 49

Pumpkin-Spiced
    Buckwheat
    Pancakes, 34
Quinoa Breakfast Power
    Bowls, 36–37
Refreshing
    Watermelon-Mint
    Smoothie, 20
Roasted Red Pepper
    and White Bean
    Shakshuka, 71
Roasted Root Vegetable
    Hash, 35
Savory Chickpea, Feta,
    and Arugula Yogurt
    Bowl, 109
Shredded Pesto Chicken
    Quinoa Bowls, 84–85
Spinach and Artichoke
    Frittata, 38
Spinach, Walnut, and
    Goat Cheese–
    Stuffed Portobello
    Mushrooms, 63
Super Green Smoothie
    Bowl, 24
Sweet Potato and Black
    Bean Burritos, 70
Sweet Potato Pie
    Smoothie, 29
Tofu Spaghetti Squash
    Pad Thai, 68–69
Triple Berry Kefir
    Smoothie, 27
Turkey-Pumpkin Chili, 47
Vanilla Matcha Latte
    Smoothie, 25
Goat cheese
    Arugula and Goat
        Cheese–Stuffed
        Chicken Breasts, 82
    Spinach, Walnut, and
        Goat Cheese–
        Stuffed Portobello
        Mushrooms, 63

Steak, Kale, and Goat
Cheese Quesadillas, 99

Goji berries, 8
Super Green Smoothie
Bowl, 24
Super Seedy No-Bake
Energy Bites, 106
Trail Mix Cookies, 111

Grains, 5–6. *See also*
specific

Grapes, 13

Greek yogurt, 11
Baked Tzatziki Pork
Loin, 96
Blackened Salmon Taco
Salad, 53
Citrus-Strawberry
Smoothie, 21
Pomegranate-Broccoli
Salad, 49
Savory Chickpea, Feta,
and Arugula Yogurt
Bowl, 109
Spicy Black Bean and
Avocado Overnight
Oats, 32
Sweet Potato Pie
Smoothie, 29

Greens, 6. *See also specific*

Grocery shopping, 14–15

H

Hemp seeds, 8
Autumn Lentil Farro
Bowls, 62
Bánh Mì Pork Farro
Bowls, 93
Citrus-Strawberry
Smoothie, 21
Crunchy Bok Choy
Slaw, 52
Lemony Blueberry-Basil
Smoothie, 22

Mongolian Beef and
Bok Choy Quinoa
Bowls, 102
Savory Chickpea, Feta,
and Arugula Yogurt
Bowl, 109
Spicy Peanut-Tofu Collard
Wraps, 66–67
Super Green Smoothie
Bowl, 24

I

Iron, 7

J

Jalapeño peppers
Bánh Mì Pork Farro
Bowls, 93
Turkey-Pumpkin Chili, 47

K

Kale, 6
Creamy Butternut
Squash and Kale
Linguine, 60
Maple-Dijon Sautéed
Kale, 54
Mushroom, Kale, and
Farro Risotto, 61
Quinoa Breakfast Power
Bowls, 36–37
Steak, Kale, and Goat
Cheese Quesadillas, 99

Kefir, 11
Triple Berry Kefir
Smoothie, 27

Kidney beans, 10
One-Pot Three-Bean
Chili, 46

Kimchi, 12

Kiwis
Super Green Smoothie
Bowl, 24

L

Legumes, 9–10. *See also*
specific

Lemons
Baked Tzatziki Pork
Loin, 96
Creamy Avocado and
Split Pea Soup, 44
Garlic-Herb Pork and
Swiss Chard
Pasta, 95
Gremolata-Stuffed
Tilapia, 76
Lemony Blueberry-Basil
Smoothie, 22
One-Pot Turkey Pasta
Primavera, 89
Pan-Seared Scallops
over Lemon-Basil
Farro, 80
Pistachio-Crusted
Salmon, 78
Raspberry-Coconut
Oatmeal Bars, 112–113
Spinach and Feta
Chickpea Burgers, 65

Lentils, 10
Autumn Lentil Farro
Bowls, 62
Lentil-Walnut Tacos, 72

Limes
Coconut-Lime Shrimp
Tacos, 79
Creamy
Pineapple-Cilantro
Smoothie, 23
Crunchy Bok Choy
Slaw, 52
Ginger-Sesame Tuna
Wraps, 77
Grilled Chicken with
Pineapple-Avocado
Salsa, 81

Limes *(Continued)*
    Grilled Chili-Lime Watermelon Wedges, 108
    Refreshing Watermelon-Mint Smoothie, 20
    Spicy Black Bean and Avocado Overnight Oats, 32
    Spicy Peanut-Tofu Collard Wraps, 66–67
    Spicy Sesame Chicken Noodle Soup, 43
    Tempeh Taco Bowls, 73
    Thai Sweet Potato Salad, 50
    Tofu Spaghetti Squash Pad Thai, 68–69

M

Macadamia nuts, 13

Magnesium, 7

Mangos
    Super Green Smoothie Bowl, 24

Matcha, 8
    Vanilla Matcha Latte Smoothie, 25

Mint
    Refreshing Watermelon-Mint Smoothie, 20

Miso, 8
    Miso Soup with Bok Choy and Tofu, 42

Mozzarella cheese
    Shredded Pesto Chicken Quinoa Bowls, 84–85
    Spinach Caprese Beef Burgers, 103

    Summer Vegetable Lasagna with Tofu Ricotta, 58–59

Mushrooms
    Beef, Mushroom, and Sweet Potato Cottage Pie, 97–98
    Mushroom, Kale, and Farro Risotto, 61
    Spinach, Walnut, and Goat Cheese-Stuffed Portobello Mushrooms, 63
    Summer Vegetable Lasagna with Tofu Ricotta, 58–59

Mussels, 10

N

Noodles
    Spicy Sesame Chicken Noodle Soup, 43

Nori seaweed
    Ginger-Sesame Tuna Wraps, 77
    Miso Soup with Bok Choy and Tofu, 42
    Savory Nori Popcorn, 107

Nutrients, 7

Nuts, 4–5. *See also specific*

O

Oats, 5
    Golden Milk Oatmeal with Toasted Pecans, 33
    Peanut Butter-Stuffed Baked Apples, 115
    Raspberry-Coconut Oatmeal Bars, 112–113
    Spicy Black Bean and Avocado Overnight Oats, 32

    Super Seedy No-Bake Energy Bites, 106
    Trail Mix Cookies, 111

One pot
    Arugula and Goat Cheese-Stuffed Chicken Breasts, 82
    Chocolate, Strawberry, and Avocado Mousse, 114
    Chocolate-Covered Cherry Smoothie, 28
    Citrus-Strawberry Smoothie, 21
    Cold Brew Mocha Smoothie, 26
    Creamy Avocado and Split Pea Soup, 44
    Creamy Butternut Squash and Kale Linguine, 60
    Creamy Pineapple-Cilantro Smoothie, 23
    Crunchy Bok Choy Slaw, 52
    Curry Vegetable Peanut Stew, 45
    Garlic-Herb Pork and Swiss Chard Pasta, 95
    Ginger Matcha "Nice" Cream, 110
    Ginger-Sesame Tuna Wraps, 77
    Lemony Blueberry-Basil Smoothie, 22
    Lentil-Walnut Tacos, 72
    Miso Soup with Bok Choy and Tofu, 42
    Mushroom, Kale, and Farro Risotto, 61
    One-Pot Three-Bean Chili, 46

One-Pot Turkey Pasta
Primavera, 89

Pomegranate-Broccoli
Salad, 49

Refreshing
Watermelon-Mint
Smoothie, 20

Roasted Red Pepper
and White Bean
Shakshuka, 71

Savory Chickpea, Feta,
and Arugula Yogurt
Bowl, 109

Savory Nori Popcorn, 107

Spicy Peanut-Tofu Collard
Wraps, 66–67

Spicy Sesame Chicken
Noodle Soup, 43

Spinach Caprese Beef
Burgers, 103

Spinach, Walnut, and
Goat Cheese–
Stuffed Portobello
Mushrooms, 63

Steak, Kale, and Goat
Cheese Quesadillas, 99

Super Green Smoothie
Bowl, 24

Super Seedy No-Bake
Energy Bites, 106

Sweet Corn Clam
Chowder, 48

Sweet Potato Pie
Smoothie, 29

Triple Berry Kefir
Smoothie, 27

Turkey-Pumpkin Chili, 47

Vanilla Matcha Latte
Smoothie, 25

Oranges, 4

Citrus-Strawberry
Smoothie, 21

Orange and Sriracha Pork
Tacos, 92

P

Pantry staples, 12

Parmesan cheese

Beef-Stuffed
Eggplant, 100

Garlic-Herb Pork and
Swiss Chard Pasta, 95

Grilled Romaine Chickpea
Caesar Salad, 51

Mushroom, Kale, and
Farro Risotto, 61

One-Pot Turkey Pasta
Primavera, 89

Shredded Pesto Chicken
Quinoa Bowls, 84–85

Spinach and Artichoke
Frittata, 38

Spinach, Walnut, and
Goat Cheese–
Stuffed Portobello
Mushrooms, 63

Summer Vegetable
Lasagna with Tofu
Ricotta, 58–59

Parsley

Garlic-Herb Pork and
Swiss Chard Pasta, 95

Gremolata-Stuffed
Tilapia, 76

Parsnips, 9

Pasta

Creamy Butternut Squash
and Kale Linguine, 60

Garlic-Herb Pork and
Swiss Chard Pasta, 95

One-Pot Turkey Pasta
Primavera, 89

Summer Vegetable
Lasagna with Tofu
Ricotta, 58–59

Peanut butter

Curry Vegetable Peanut
Stew, 45

Peanut Butter–Stuffed
Baked Apples, 115

Spicy Peanut-Tofu Collard
Wraps, 66–67

Super Seedy No-Bake
Energy Bites, 106

Thai Sweet Potato
Salad, 50

Trail Mix Cookies, 111

Peanuts, 10

Thai Sweet Potato
Salad, 50

Tofu Spaghetti Squash
Pad Thai, 68–69

Peas, 10. *See also* **Split peas**

Pecans, 4

Crispy Pecan-Baked
Chicken, 83

Golden Milk Oatmeal
with Toasted
Pecans, 33

Peppers. *See* **Bell peppers;**
Jalapeño peppers;
Serrano peppers

Pineapple, 4

Creamy
Pineapple-Cilantro
Smoothie, 23

Grilled Chicken with
Pineapple-Avocado
Salsa, 81

Pineapple Curry Turkey
Burgers, 88

Pinto beans

One-Pot Three-Bean
Chili, 46

Turkey-Pumpkin Chili, 47

Pistachios, 4–5

Pistachio-Crusted
Salmon, 78

Pomegranates, 4

Pomegranate-Broccoli
Salad, 49

Popcorn

Savory Nori Popcorn, 107

Pork

Baked Tzatziki Pork
Loin, 96

Bánh Mì Pork Farro
Bowls, 93

Garlic-Herb Pork and
Swiss Chard
Pasta, 95

Orange and Sriracha Pork
Tacos, 92

Oven-Roasted Pork
Chops with Apples and
Walnuts, 94

Potatoes, 9

Roasted Root Vegetable
Hash, 35

Sweet Corn Clam
Chowder, 48

Pumpkin purée

Pumpkin-Spiced
Buckwheat
Pancakes, 34

Turkey-Pumpkin
Chili, 47

Pumpkin seeds, 5

Autumn Lentil Farro
Bowls, 62

Super Seedy No-Bake
Energy Bites, 106

Trail Mix Cookies, 111

Q

Quinoa, 6

Mongolian Beef and
Bok Choy Quinoa
Bowls, 102

Quinoa Breakfast Power
Bowls, 36–37

Shredded Pesto Chicken
Quinoa Bowls, 84–85

Tempeh Taco Bowls, 73

R

Radishes, 9

Baked Radishes with
Balsamic Vinegar, 55

Bánh Mì Pork Farro
Bowls, 93

Raspberries

Raspberry-Coconut
Oatmeal Bars, 112–113

Recipes, about, 16–17

Refrigerator staples, 12

Rice. *See* Brown rice

Ricotta cheese

Ricotta, Blackberry, and
Arugula Flatbreads, 64

Romaine lettuce, 6

Blackened Salmon Taco
Salad, 53

Grilled Romaine Chickpea
Caesar Salad, 51

Tempeh Taco Bowls, 73

Roots and tubers, 9.
See also specific

S

Sage

Creamy Butternut Squash
and Kale Linguine, 60

Salads

Blackened Salmon Taco
Salad, 53

Crunchy Bok Choy
Slaw, 52

Grilled Romaine Chickpea
Caesar Salad, 51

Pomegranate-Broccoli
Salad, 49

Thai Sweet Potato
Salad, 50

Salmon, 10

Blackened Salmon Taco
Salad, 53

Pistachio-Crusted
Salmon, 78

Sardines, 10

Sauerkraut, 12

Scallops, 11

Pan-Seared Scallops over
Lemon-Basil Farro, 80

**Seafood, 10–11. *See also
specific***

Seeds, 5. *See also specific*

Serrano peppers

Thai Basil Beef–Stuffed
Sweet Potatoes, 101

Sesame seeds, 5

Ginger-Sesame Tuna
Wraps, 77

Spicy Sesame Chicken
Noodle Soup, 43

Shrimp, 11

Coconut-Lime Shrimp
Tacos, 79

Smoothies

Chocolate-Covered
Cherry Smoothie, 28

Citrus-Strawberry
Smoothie, 21

Cold Brew Mocha
Smoothie, 26

Creamy
Pineapple-Cilantro
Smoothie, 23

Lemony Blueberry-Basil
Smoothie, 22

Refreshing
Watermelon-Mint
Smoothie, 20

Super Green Smoothie
Bowl, 24

Sweet Potato Pie
Smoothie, 29

Triple Berry Kefir
Smoothie, 27

Vanilla Matcha Latte
Smoothie, 25

Snacks, 14

Grilled Chili-Lime
Watermelon
Wedges, 108

Raspberry-Coconut
Oatmeal Bars, 112–113

Savory Chickpea, Feta,
and Arugula Yogurt
Bowl, 109

Savory Nori Popcorn, 107

Super Seedy No-Bake
Energy Bites, 106

Soups

Creamy Avocado and
Split Pea Soup, 44

Miso Soup with Bok Choy
and Tofu, 42

One-Pot Three-Bean
Chili, 46

Spicy Sesame Chicken
Noodle Soup, 43

Sweet Corn Clam
Chowder, 48

Turkey-Pumpkin Chili, 47

Spices, 14

Spinach, 6

Autumn Lentil Farro
Bowls, 62

Beef-Stuffed
Eggplant, 100

Creamy
Pineapple-Cilantro
Smoothie, 23

Curry Vegetable Peanut
Stew, 45

Greek Turkey and
Barley-Stuffed
Peppers, 86–87

Spinach, Walnut, and
Goat Cheese–
Stuffed Portobello
Mushrooms, 63

Spinach and Artichoke
Frittata, 38

Spinach and Feta
Chickpea Burgers, 65

Spinach Caprese Beef
Burgers, 103

Summer Vegetable
Lasagna with Tofu
Ricotta, 58–59

Super Green Smoothie
Bowl, 24

Sweet Potato and Black
Bean Burritos, 70

Spirulina, 8

Split peas

Creamy Avocado and
Split Pea Soup, 44

Squash. *See also* **Zucchini**

Creamy Butternut
Squash and Kale
Linguine, 60

Tofu Spaghetti Squash
Pad Thai, 68–69

Strawberries, 4

Chocolate, Strawberry,
and Avocado
Mousse, 114

Citrus-Strawberry
Smoothie, 21

Refreshing
Watermelon-Mint
Smoothie, 20

Super Green Smoothie
Bowl, 24

Triple Berry Kefir
Smoothie, 27

Sunflower seeds, 13

Superfoods

about, 2–3

fruits, 3–4

grains, 5–6

nutrient sources, 7

nuts and seeds, 4–5

other, 11–12

roots and tubers, 9

seafood, 10–11

specialty, 8

Supplements, 3

Sweet potatoes, 9

Beef, Mushroom, and
Sweet Potato Cottage
Pie, 97–98

Curry Vegetable Peanut
Stew, 45

Quinoa Breakfast Power
Bowls, 36–37

Sweet Potato and Black
Bean Burritos, 70

Sweet Potato Pie
Smoothie, 29

Thai Basil Beef-Stuffed
Sweet Potatoes, 101

Thai Sweet Potato
Salad, 50

Swiss chard, 6

Garlic-Herb Pork and
Swiss Chard Pasta, 95

T

Tacos

Blackened Salmon
Taco Salad, 53

Coconut-Lime Shrimp
Tacos, 79

Lentil-Walnut Tacos, 72

Orange and Sriracha Pork
Tacos, 92

Tempeh Taco Bowls, 73

Tempeh

Tempeh Taco Bowls, 73

30 minutes

Arugula and Goat
Cheese–Stuffed
Chicken Breasts, 82

Bánh Mì Pork Farro
Bowls, 93

Blackened Salmon Taco
Salad, 53

30 minutes *(Continued)*

Chocolate, Strawberry, and Avocado Mousse, 114

Chocolate-Covered Cherry Smoothie, 28

Citrus-Strawberry Smoothie, 21

Coconut-Lime Shrimp Tacos, 79

Cold Brew Mocha Smoothie, 26

Creamy Butternut Squash and Kale Linguine, 60

Creamy Pineapple-Cilantro Smoothie, 23

Crispy Pecan-Baked Chicken, 83

Curry Vegetable Peanut Stew, 45

Garlic-Herb Pork and Swiss Chard Pasta, 95

Ginger Matcha "Nice" Cream, 110

Ginger-Sesame Tuna Wraps, 77

Golden Milk Oatmeal with Toasted Pecans, 33

Gremolata-Stuffed Tilapia, 76

Grilled Chicken with Pineapple-Avocado Salsa, 81

Grilled Chili-Lime Watermelon Wedges, 108

Grilled Romaine Chickpea Caesar Salad, 51

Lemony Blueberry-Basil Smoothie, 22

Lentil-Walnut Tacos, 72

Maple-Dijon Sautéed Kale, 54

Miso Soup with Bok Choy and Tofu, 42

One-Pot Three-Bean Chili, 46

One-Pot Turkey Pasta Primavera, 89

Orange and Sriracha Pork Tacos, 92

Pan-Seared Scallops over Lemon-Basil Farro, 80

Pineapple Curry Turkey Burgers, 88

Pistachio-Crusted Salmon, 78

Pumpkin-Spiced Buckwheat Pancakes, 34

Quinoa Breakfast Power Bowls, 36–37

Refreshing Watermelon-Mint Smoothie, 20

Ricotta, Blackberry, and Arugula Flatbreads, 64

Roasted Red Pepper and White Bean Shakshuka, 71

Savory Chickpea, Feta, and Arugula Yogurt Bowl, 109

Savory Nori Popcorn, 107

Shredded Pesto Chicken Quinoa Bowls, 84–85

Spicy Peanut-Tofu Collard Wraps, 66–67

Spicy Sesame Chicken Noodle Soup, 43

Spinach and Artichoke Frittata, 38

Spinach and Feta Chickpea Burgers, 65

Spinach Caprese Beef Burgers, 103

Spinach, Walnut, and Goat Cheese–Stuffed Portobello Mushrooms, 63

Steak, Kale, and Goat Cheese Quesadillas, 99

Super Green Smoothie Bowl, 24

Super Seedy No-Bake Energy Bites, 106

Sweet Corn Clam Chowder, 48

Sweet Potato and Black Bean Burritos, 70

Sweet Potato Pie Smoothie, 29

Thai Basil Beef-Stuffed Sweet Potatoes, 101

Trail Mix Cookies, 111

Triple Berry Kefir Smoothie, 27

Turkey-Pumpkin Chili, 47

Vanilla Matcha Latte Smoothie, 25

Tilapia

Gremolata-Stuffed Tilapia, 76

Tofu, 11

Miso Soup with Bok Choy and Tofu, 42

Spicy Peanut-Tofu Collard Wraps, 66–67

Summer Vegetable Lasagna with Tofu Ricotta, 58–59

Tofu Spaghetti Squash Pad Thai, 68–69

Tomatoes

Blackened Salmon Taco Salad, 53

Curry Vegetable Peanut Stew, 45

Greek Turkey and Barley–Stuffed Peppers, 86–87

One-Pot Three-Bean
Chili, 46

Roasted Red Pepper
and White Bean
Shakshuka, 71

Shredded Pesto Chicken
Quinoa Bowls, 84–85

Spinach Caprese Beef
Burgers, 103

Tuna, 11

Ginger-Sesame Tuna
Wraps, 77

Turkey

Greek Turkey and Barley-
Stuffed Peppers, 86–87

One-Pot Turkey Pasta
Primavera, 89

Pineapple Curry Turkey
Burgers, 88

Turkey-Pumpkin Chili, 47

Turmeric, 8

V

Vegan

Autumn Lentil Farro
Bowls, 62

Baked Radishes with
Balsamic Vinegar, 55

Chocolate, Strawberry,
and Avocado
Mousse, 114

Chocolate-Covered
Cherry Smoothie, 28

Cold Brew Mocha
Smoothie, 26

Creamy Avocado and
Split Pea Soup, 44

Creamy Butternut Squash
and Kale Linguine, 60

Curry Vegetable Peanut
Stew, 45

Ginger Matcha "Nice"
Cream, 110

Grilled Chili-Lime
Watermelon
Wedges, 108

Lemony Blueberry-Basil
Smoothie, 22

Lentil-Walnut Tacos, 72

Maple-Dijon Sautéed
Kale, 54

Miso Soup with Bok Choy
and Tofu, 42

One-Pot Three-Bean
Chili, 46

Peanut Butter-Stuffed
Baked Apples, 115

Raspberry-Coconut
Oatmeal Bars, 112–113

Refreshing
Watermelon-Mint
Smoothie, 20

Roasted Root Vegetable
Hash, 35

Savory Nori Popcorn, 107

Spicy Peanut-Tofu Collard
Wraps, 66–67

Super Green Smoothie
Bowl, 24

Super Seedy No-Bake
Energy Bites, 106

Tempeh Taco Bowls, 73

Trail Mix Cookies, 111

Vegetables. *See also*
specific

Beef, Mushroom, and
Sweet Potato Cottage
Pie, 97–98

Vegetarian. *See also* **Vegan**

Citrus-Strawberry
Smoothie, 21

Creamy
Pineapple-Cilantro
Smoothie, 23

Crunchy Bok Choy
Slaw, 52

Golden Milk Oatmeal with
Toasted Pecans, 33

Grilled Romaine
Chickpea Caesar
Salad, 51

Mushroom, Kale, and
Farro Risotto, 61

Pomegranate-Broccoli
Salad, 49

Pumpkin-Spiced
Buckwheat
Pancakes, 34

Quinoa Breakfast Power
Bowls, 36–37

Ricotta, Blackberry, and
Arugula Flatbreads, 64

Roasted Red Pepper
and White Bean
Shakshuka, 71

Savory Chickpea, Feta,
and Arugula Yogurt
Bowl, 109

Spicy Black Bean and
Avocado Overnight
Oats, 32

Spinach and Artichoke
Frittata, 38

Spinach and Feta
Chickpea Burgers, 65

Spinach, Walnut, and
Goat Cheese-
Stuffed Portobello
Mushrooms, 63

Summer Vegetable
Lasagna with Tofu
Ricotta, 58–59

Sweet Potato and Black
Bean Burritos, 70

Sweet Potato Pie
Smoothie, 29

Thai Sweet Potato
Salad, 50

Tofu Spaghetti Squash
Pad Thai, 68–69

Vegetarian *(Continued)*

Triple Berry Kefir
Smoothie, 27

Vanilla Matcha Latte
Smoothie, 25

Vitamin B$_{12}$, 7

Vitamin D, 7

Walnuts, 5

Autumn Lentil Farro
Bowls, 62

Lentil-Walnut Tacos, 72

Oven-Roasted Pork
Chops with Apples
and Walnuts, 94

Pomegranate-Broccoli
Salad, 49

Pumpkin-Spiced
Buckwheat
Pancakes, 34

Spinach, Walnut, and
Goat Cheese-
Stuffed Portobello
Mushrooms, 63

Trail Mix Cookies, 111

Watermelon, 4

Grilled Chili-Lime
Watermelon
Wedges, 108

Refreshing Watermelon-
Mint Smoothie, 20

White beans

Roasted Red Pepper
and White Bean
Shakshuka, 71

Wraps. *See also* **Tacos**

Ginger-Sesame Tuna
Wraps, 77

Spicy Peanut-Tofu Collard
Wraps, 66–67

Steak, Kale, and Goat
Cheese Quesadillas, 99

Sweet Potato and Black
Bean Burritos, 70

Yogurt. *See* **Greek yogurt**

Z

Zucchini

One-Pot Turkey Pasta
Primavera, 89

Summer Vegetable
Lasagna with Tofu
Ricotta, 58–59

Acknowledgments

I would first like to thank Diane and Jerry for their support and encouragement every step of the way. This book is possible because of you. Thanks to my parents for letting me carve my own path, even if neither they nor I knew where I was going; my friends for being my loudest and proudest fans; and Rob, my love—how grateful I am to have you by my side through it all. Life is better with you.

About the Author

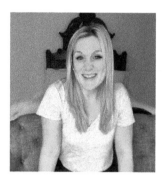

Emily Cooper, RD, was born and raised in New Hampshire and is a registered dietitian, nationally recognized food and nutrition expert, and award-winning recipe developer. She shares quick and healthy recipes on her website, Sinful Nutrition (SinfulNutrition.com), where she's passionate about showing that eating healthier doesn't have to be boring, expensive, or difficult.

CPSIA information can be obtained
at www.ICGtesting.com
Printed in the USA
BVHW061753020120
568213BV00001B/1